SURGERY - PROCEDURES, COMPLICATIONS, AND RESULTS

PRINCIPLES OF RESEARCH

FROM IDEA TO PUBLICATION

SURGERY - PROCEDURES, COMPLICATIONS, AND RESULTS

Additional books in this series can be found on Nova's website under the Series tab.

Additional e-books in this series can be found on Nova's website under the e-book tab.

SURGERY - PROCEDURES, COMPLICATIONS, AND RESULTS

PRINCIPLES OF RESEARCH

FROM IDEA TO PUBLICATION

LUIS H. TOLEDO-PEREYRA
EDITOR

New York

For permission to use material from this book please contact us:
Telephone 631-231-7269; Fax 631-231-8175
Web Site: http://www.novapublishers.com

Library of Congress Cataloging-in-Publication Data

ISBN: 978-1-62417-968-6

Library of Congress Control Number: 2012956450

Published by Nova Science Publishers, Inc. † New York

To each one of the medical students, residents and faculty who are determined to utilize research in the advancement of medical care for their own patients.

CONTENTS

A Note of Recognition

Many chapters in this book have appeared before in the *Journal of Investigative Surgery*. We appreciate the permission given by *Informa USA* to reproduce them. Modification and additions were incorporated to previous publications.

Preface

CREATING THE MEDICINE OF THE FUTURE

Luis H. Toledo-Pereyra
Western Michigan University School of Medicine,
Michigan State University College of Human Medicine,
Michigan State University College of Osteopathic Medicine,
Kalamazoo, MI, US

Research is essential for improving clinical practice and for advancing the optimal care of patients in need [1, 2]. Without research we cannot offer patients the best available therapy. We must then learn research at a minimum to be at pace with the medical developments of the times and we must utilize research under ideal conditions to create the medicine of the future.

Creating the medicine of the future is not that simple, but in a different way is our responsibility since patient care is at the core of the physician's professional practice. Research will give us the fundamental key to formulate and develop the medicine of the future. The medicine than can help our patients!

Creating the medicine of the future is particularly challenging even though circumscribed to the area of medical concern. Research offers the opportunity to resolve the demands of medical progress. When research is used appropriately the better understanding and treatment of disease becomes more attainable.

CREATING THE MEDICINE OF THE FUTURE IS AN OBLIGATION

Physicians, surgeons or any other specialist or professional in healthcare have the unique obligation of improving the well-being of their patients. This goal can be best reached through the virtues of a well-planned and fully organized research endeavor.

Research brings knowledge to patient care and as such would permit advancing the cure of patients seeking the physician's help. Research within this context is curing and therefore, advancing medicine or in other words creating the medicine of the future.

Research means progress. Research establishes the difference between systematic analysis of healthcare and practical approach to the practice of medicine. Research is clearly the motor behind creating the medicine of the future.

RESEARCH IS THE MEDICINE OF THE FUTURE

It is clear, at least to many of us, that without research the medicine of the future would not exist. We have many examples that prove this assumption. In this regard, it is not easy to know where to start since we could go from the advances attributed to the tiny molecule of acetylsalicylic acid (aspirin) in inflammation, cardiovascular medicine and cancer to its original effect initially observed as potent analgesic [3].

On the other hand, we could consider very complex biological molecules in the likes of Vemurafenib which after extensive molecular biology laboratory work demonstrated to be very effective for late stages melanoma [4]. The previous two examples demonstrate how the medicine of the future can only be created with thoughtful and carefully planned research. Analyzing old compounds and/or introducing new molecules will permit to advance the medicine of the future, the medicine that will save the lives of a great number of patients.

PREPARING TO CREATE THE MEDICINE OF THE FUTURE

It appears clear that the medicine of the future will only respond to carefully orchestrated research. That to make advances worth mentioning our physicians and healthcare personnel must engage themselves on a well-crafted research plan. That placing research at the forefront would be not only good but imperative. And, that within the education of physicians, emphasis should be placed on the teaching of the most current research practices that might permit a steady progress on the best results of medical care.

Preparing not only faculty and residents is important but the education of medical students is fundamental when considering the medicine of the future. The research education of younger generations should create the optimal environment for moving toward the medicine being practiced today.

In conclusion, learning and applying the best principles of research to medical practice will increase the possibilities of creating the medicine of the future.

REFERENCES

[1] Toledo-Pereyra LH. Importance of Research in Toledo-Pereyra, LH, *Principles of Research. From Idea to Publication*. Chapter 1, pp 17-23, 2013.

[2] Dormitorio B, Flikkema R, Toledo AH, Toledo-Pereyra LH. Statistical Analysis in Toledo-Pereyra LH, *Principles of Research. From Idea to Publication*. Chapter 7, pp 53-69, 2013.

[3] Jeffreys D. *Aspirin. The Story of a Wonder Drug*. Bloomsbury, USA, 2004.

[4] Chapman PB, Hauschild A, Robert C., et al. Improved Survival with Vemurafenib in Melanoma with BRAF V600E Mutation. *N Eng J Med;* 364:2507-16, 2011.

Introduction

Motivating a New Generation of Researchers

Luis H. Toledo-Pereyra
Western Michigan University School of Medicine,
Michigan State University College of Human Medicine,
Michigan State University College of Osteopathic Medicine,
Kalamazoo, MI, US

Advancing research to high levels of awareness and accomplishment is closely dependent on motivating the new generation of researchers. These researchers will most likely bring an enriched spirit of innovation and development so necessary to move ahead the research agenda.

The question is how to motivate the new generation of researchers? what plan should we use as the most effective for the future generation of physicians? What approach should take us to a more constant advancement of research ideas and results?

In motivating a new generation of researchers we must include three important areas: one, the demonstration of the benefit of research; two, the evaluation of the research strategy, and three, the clarification of how research was conceived.

Motivating a new generation of researchers will not be simple unless emphasis is directed at research results and its applicability to clinical care. This is considered to be translational research of so much interest these days [1, 2].

Characterization and decisive support of the new researcher should be a focus of interest when motivating the new generation of physicians who would like to be active participants of the research academic enterprise.

The new researcher is someone who is committed to finding the answers to the clinical problems facing our patients today. From little problems that appear at any level of patient interaction to major developments confronting the patient's lives, the new researcher is dedicated to encountering solutions for these simple or complex problems. The new researcher is aware of critical medical situations and does not chide away from them. The new researcher is dedicated to protecting and helping patients by studying and advancing the knowledge and required for overcoming disease.

In short, we need to motivate and maintain the spirit alive of the new generation of researchers since only by motivating them we can develop and maximize the best research possible.

References

[1] Coppens M, Eikeboom JW, Gustafsson D, et al. Translation Success Stories: Development of Direct Thrombin Inhibitors. *Circ. Res.* 14;920-9, 2012.

[2] Hayes H, Burge S. Creating a Practice Based Research Network From Scratch; Where do I Begin? *Prog. Community Health Partners*. 6:369-80, 2012.

SECTION I
PRINCIPLES OF RESEARCH

In: Principles of Research
Editor: Luis H. Toledo-Pereyra
ISBN: 978-1-62417-968-6

Chapter 1

IMPORTANCE OF RESEARCH

Luis H. Toledo-Pereyra
Western Michigan University School of Medicine,
Michigan State University College of Human Medicine,
Michigan State University College of Osteopathic Medicine,
Kalamazoo, MI, US

This is not a long chapter, neither it is unimportant, but its significance requires conciseness and well-defined attention. The importance of research is obvious for many but some still have questions about the direct application of research to clinical medicine. We focus on this chapter on the demonstrated utility of research, even though this topic of the importance of research it does not need introduction since we all most likely agree that research represents the real backbone of medicine and surgery.

Without research the advancement of medicine and surgery is not possible. To reach progress can only be seen on the dedicated pursue of research. Research is at the forefront of patient care whether medical or surgical. Centuries of creative research have opened the doors to new medical and surgical frontiers that before would not have been feasible. Medical and surgical sciences would not have climbed to the heights we know today without the perseverance and insistence of research. Research has been the driving force introducing new directions on the improvement of medicine and surgery.

Research gives us information and more precise knowledge, elements of new and innovative findings, and possibilities for improved treatments.

Without research we would not be able to help the thousands or more precisely the more than millions of patients who have benefited so far when conquering the evolution of disease affecting the world. Without research, stagnation in medicine and surgery would rein at all times. Without research, patients and doctors would not have the same knowledge capabilities in treating maladies that we currently treat. Research, then, is essential to medicine and surgery.

Discovery and validation represent two of the most critical developments signaling the importance of research. On the one side, discovery brings new findings, new treatments, new surgical procedures, and/or new device manufacturing and utilization. Whereas, on the other hand, validation is a confirmatory process that permits full demonstration that the findings, treatments, procedures, and/or devices are real and worth applying in practice. Both of these elements, discovery and validation are necessary to categorize and define research in a more appropriate manner, a complete manner. Research depends on discovery and validation to exert its complete and fully intended effect. Alone, research would have limited influence.

The importance of research is magnified by the incredible discoveries introduced into the medical and surgical sciences. Consider the diabetic patient who lives for decades without succumbing to the effects of waste and metabolic derangement because of the lack of insulin, or the ominous death sentence associated with the ravages of end-stage liver failure because of the absence of a new liver to be transplanted. One can readily see how research opened up a glorious era of treatment never seen before. Today diabetics get insulin, liver failure patients get liver transplants, Alzheimer's patients get improved medical treatments, vascular disease patients receive prompt and effective surgical attention, cancer patients, as hard as it might be to believe, more frequently now than ever before achieve cure. And these are only a few of many such significant advances. Of course, there is no parallel in the history of medicine, surgery, or the scientific fields to the advances realized by medicine and surgery during the 20th century [1]. And, by all means and as repetitive as it might be, research was a constant companion to all of these extraordinary changes.

Research is the guiding light for innovators and discoverers who want to advance the understanding of disease in the medical and surgical world [2]. Research equals knowledge, which at the same time can heal patients who initially had no treatment for their illnesses. Research is the force behind investigators who otherwise could not progress in their march toward defining the best paths to health and cure. Research is the well-defined structure that needs to be moved ahead to find solutions for those who were once considered to have incurable problems.

The word research is not that old since originated only five centuries ago (3). It came from the French *"rechercher,"* which means *"to search"* [3]. As time progressed, the meaning of the word eventually became associated with science and specifically with what we call *scientific research*. Even though the two words, science and research, are sometimes closely associated, in reality they have different connotations since the first one is a general discipline and the second one a way to study that discipline.

The scientific tradition goes back to the Greeks in the fifth century BC and later, it moved to Aristotle (384-322 BC) when he excelled in the fourth century BC by introducing the scientific method and contributing to the philosophical movement of Empiricism. In addition, Aristotle conceived deductive reasoning particularly with the use of syllogisms [4]. Others followed, such as the Arabs, Roger Bacon (1213-1294), Galileo Galilei (1564-1642), Rene Descartes (1596-1650), Isaac Newton (1642-1727), and many more who stood out among many noted scientists and contributors to the science of their times. Research was beginning to create its own presence as science advanced to levels that were better understood although unpredictable. With the knowledge encountered by the scientific method, research proceeded to further enhance the information and discovery still missing in several accounts of the scientific process.

It is of no surprise that research has been the main engine for the medical developments encountered by physicians and surgeons of our times. Research constitutes the only solution to continuing the best progress we need in this new century. One could summarize this chapter by saying that research equals advancement that at the same time equals better health for all. Perhaps, this last statement epitomizes the goals and aspirations of research.

REFERENCES

[1] Friedman M, Friedland GW, *Medicine 10 Greatest Discoveries*. New Haven, CT: Yale University Press; 1998.

[2] Toledo-Pereyra LH. *Innovation and Discovery on Surgery, History and Humanities*. Austin, TX: Landes Bioscience; 2009.

[3] *The American Heritage Dictionary of the English Language*. New York: Houghton Mifflin; 2009, Available at: Resaerch.Dictionary.Com, accessed August 31, 2009.

[4] *History of Scientific Method*. Available at: Wikipedia.com, accessed August 31, 2009.

MEDICAL STUDENT PERSPECTIVE

Nicholas Ahn
Michigan State University College of Human Medicine,
Kalamazoo Campus, Kalamazoo, MI, US

The Importance of Research in Clinical Medicine

Antibiotics, Insulin, the Human Genome Project. Without clinical research, none of these major advances would have been possible. While modern medicine allows us to do many miracles, none of them would exist without some of the most basic theories we take for granted. We take for granted now that children everywhere get standard vaccinations that prevent the likes of polio, rabies, mumps, and smallpox. However, in the early 1800s, these were terrible, debilitating diseases that often took the lives of all people, rich and poor. We also take for granted the knowledge that germs reside everywhere and cause disease in people. This theory allows us to prevent disease through sanitation and antibiotics. Again, such a simple theory has probably prevented millions of deaths, but was relatively unknown until the work of clinical scientists.

One of the earliest and most powerful examples of this concept comes from the work of country doctor Edward Jenner. Jenner was fascinated by the wives' tale that milkmaids did not contract smallpox. He noted that milkmaids did seem to get cowpox, a weaker version of smallpox, but did not get smallpox itself. He also saw that milkmaids got a number or blisters filled with pus on their hands. Jenner concluded that something in the pus must somehow prevent the transmission of smallpox. The doctor tested his theory by injecting some of the pus from a milkmaid's cowpox blisters into a young boy named James Phipps. Through sequential vaccination and then deliberately injecting smallpox into the boy, Jenner proved that smallpox could indeed be prevented through vaccination. It was a brilliant discovery that formed the basis for another famous scientist's work.

The germ theory also comes from an example of research that eventually led to groundbreaking work in medicine. French chemist and microbiologist Louis Pasteur studied beer, wine, pebrine, and other diseases on his way to creating his famous theories. In 1856, Pasteur was commissioned by an alcohol manufacturer to discovery the reason for vats of fermented beer turning sour. Using a microscopic Pasteur looked at samples of the beer and discovered tiny micro-organisms in the beer. He theorized that these micro-organisms were causing the beer to go sour. He further continued work into other liquids such as milk and wine. Through this work, he became even more convinced of his theory and elaborated upon it, announcing that he believed that microbes in the air were contaminating these liquids. Though he was ridiculed, he eventually proved that his theory was correct beyond any shadow of a doubt.

In addition, Pasteur took this work further in an investigation of a plague affecting the silk worm industry. In only a year, Pasteur discovered that the disease was caused by another living organism and postulated that humans as well as the beer and silk worms could be affected by microbes. He then took this theory further by trying to create a vaccine for chicken cholera, a disease that plagued poultry farmers. Though he knew of the work done by Edward Jenner, he did not know the theory and thus was clueless as to how to continue with his work.

In 1880, he discovered the vaccine by accident when a member of his research team inoculated some chickens with an old cholera culture. Through further research, Pasteur eventually discovered the key to a vaccine – use a weakened version of the microbe that caused the disease. He continued with this theory to successfully create vaccines for anthrax in animals, and as a crowning achievement, successfully immunized the first human to rabies.

These men lay down the groundwork for our current vaccination campaigns. These vaccines have prevented hundreds of thousands of infections and completely eliminated the disease of smallpox. Without research like this into some of the basic sciences, modern medicine would never have had a framework it does today to create and further elaborate upon these discoveries and apply them to curing diseases. The work of Edward Jenner and Louis Pasteur, along with many other scientists through the ages, have given us a gift that truly keeps on giving – the basis for clinical medical knowledge.

References

BBC. (n.d.) Louis Pasteur. BBC – History – Louis Pasteur. Retrieved 1/23/12 from *http://www.bbc.co.uk/history/historic_figures/pasteur_louis.shtml.*

Cohn, David (1999) The Life and Times of Louis Pasteur. Lab Explorers. Retrieved 1/23/12 from *http://www.labexplorer.com/louis pasteur.htm.*

Pasteur, Louis. (n.d.) On the Extension of the Germ Theory to the Etiology of Certain Common Diseases. Pasteur's paper on the Germ Theory. Retrieved 1/23/12 from *http://biotech.law.lsu.edu/cphl/history/articles/pasteur.htm#top.*

Pasteur, Louis. (n.d.) The Germ Theory and its Applications to Medicine and Surgery. Pastuer's paper on the Germ Theory. Retrieved 1/23/12 from *http://biotech.law.lsu.edu/cphl/history/articles/pasteur.htm#top.*

Pasteur, Louis. (n.d.) The Physiological Theory of Fermentation. Pasteur's Paper on the Germ Theory. Retrieved 1/23/12 from *http://biotach.law.lsu.edu/cphl/history/articles/pasteurlhtm#top.*

Riedel, Stefan. (2005) *Edward Jenner and the history of smallpox and vaccination.* Baylor Uni Med Cent, 18(1):21-25.

Medical Student Perspective

Nagarajan Muthu

Michigan State University College of Human Medicine,
Kalamazoo Campus, Kalamazoo, MI, US

The Importance of Research in Clinical Medicine

Medicine is the science and art of healing people. It is a constantly evolving field and throughout history, its evolution has underscored major human accomplishments in every field. Without evolution in medicine, evolution in other fields, from astronomy to zoology, would have been limited, because human life itself is limited. Therefore, it is imperative to our species' success and growth to constantly explore new possibilities and advancement in the betterment of human health.

This is only possible with continued research and application of new knowledge in healing people. It is the cornerstone to all our advancements thus far and without it, not only our level of knowledge and medical care will be stagnant, but actually start falling in its quality. Disease and disease causing agents are becoming more elusive, microbes are becoming more resistant, and as it is apparent from wars to bioterrorism, our species has a special talent in discovering new ways to harm ourselves. Therefore, if not for the advancement of human life, it is necessary to be constantly engaged in medical research to at least sustain the level of our quality of life [1].

Medical research, furthermore, represents the inherent curiosity and aptitude for understanding our natural world around us that is essential for the formation of a good physician. In fact, from my personal experience, I will argue that for most medical students, a curiosity and a basic aptitude for science at a very early age was definitely a very important reason for them to pursue medicine as a career. Compassion to help those in need was a byproduct of development that comes with time, as one matures. But that curiosity to learn, it predates the desire to help others, and it is almost as if it is our first love that made us pursue medicine.

Therefore, physicians became physicians for two reasons: desire to help others who need care and curiosity of our natural world. If they lack any one of the two, they then are not able to deliver appropriate and adequate care. For competency in knowledge without compassion and compassion without competency both represent an inadequate physician.

REFERENCES

[1] Groninger, H., Kirkpatrick, J. Putting it all together: the art and science of medicine. *Virtual Mentor*. July 2006, Volume 8, Number 7:452-458.

In: Principles of Research
Editor: Luis H. Toledo-Pereyra
ISBN: 978-1-62417-968-6

Chapter 2

Interest in Research

Luis H. Toledo-Pereyra
Western Michigan University School of Medicine,
Michigan State University College of Human Medicine,
Michigan State University College of Osteopathic Medicine,
Kalamazoo, MI, US

Interest in research is the basis for beginning a successful career in the practice of medicine. On one side, being interested in research and practicing it would permit us to realize the most of our goals and aspirations to help our patients on the solution of their illnesses. On the other side, interest in research will give us a great satisfaction to advance the cure of difficult medical or problems. Of the important elements attributed to a good medical or surgical researcher, a demonstrated interest in research is by itself of unique value since without interest nothing happens [1-5]. Interest in research creates the necessary impetus to develop and promote an effective research idea.

This chapter deals with the interest in research and the research results used today as the basis to benefit research in the clinical sciences and patient care. Furthermore, bringing the importance of research interest into medical and surgical staff meetings represents the best way to position its prominence among all attendees. Knowing that research is the basis for evidence-based medicine makes it obvious that having interest in research would facilitate the understanding and application of evidence-based principles. In this regard, then, interest in research becomes of paramount importance.

How Can the Interest in Research Be Encouraged?

For those medical students, residents and faculty who are interested in research, half of the battle is won since there is no need to prove to them the value of research and its associated results. Our goal is to convince and prepare a good plan for those who have an interest in research. This is the group to whom we must present our most persuasive arguments and from whom we need to secure participation.

Probably the best way to encourage interest in medical and surgical research is to demonstrate the best examples and special advantages of research, which in history have benefitted thousands and sometimes millions of patients. Their diseases would not have been conquered without an effective research process. The opportunity to improve medical care and influence medical and surgical progress, we believe, is only through a dedicated research program. A program that can be clear and offer results!

Results in research is the main step in gathering the attention of non-believers. Interest in research is vital if one is to promote better results in clinical medicine and surgery. Without research it is not possible to reach meaningful results. Interest in research is behind all advances so far obtained in medicine and surgery.

Even if diseases can only be controlled or improved and not cured by using research skills and knowledge, research equals improvement and betterment for suffering patients. In this regard, interest would be generated because of the clear positive message of patient improvement after using the findings of research as the best current medicine for these poorly healing individuals.

How Can the Interest in Research be Maintained?

I think this is an important question. In this regard, let's assume that interest has been generated through direct evidence of the results obtained. In this case, how can we maintain the interest in research? With improved results? With improved patient satisfaction? With advancing patient care and understanding better the process of disease? Who knows exactly but these previously mentioned elements are very important.

I put forward that we should be able to maintain the interest, first, by introducing the benefits reached through research, and second, by the desire of advancing the science of medicine and/or surgery and patient care. At this point, we have fully reached the primary goals of medical and surgical research, that is, to promote the knowledge and understanding of the medical and surgical sciences.

The development of continuous ways to overcome the challenges of patients' diseases not yet dominated by current clinical practice would maintain the interest in research because of the opportunities to improve patient care and final results. There is no question, in my mind, that better results will be conducive to more interest and renewed desire to do research or, minimally, to think about research.

Another way to maintain the interest in research is by permitting those potentially incredulous individuals to offer suggestions that might be of help to patients suffering from incurable problems or diseases. And those suggestions can be brought to the forefront of patient care as a possibly new development that could help patients in the future.

How Can a Good Plan for Enhancing the Interest in Research of Students, Residents and Faculty be Offered?

Interest in research can only be enhanced if worthwhile projects are pursued and well-presented at many of the staff meetings currently taking place at the institution. The practicality of all clinical cases discussed, as important as it is, should also be used to promote interest in research. Indeed, research might be the best ally to the clinical sciences in obtaining the best results possible.

Medical students and residents need to receive a good image of the importance of research in medicine so they become more engaged in the research approach to medicine. After all, research is evidence-based medicine, which is much proposed and supported throughout our medical education system.

Encouraging medical students and residents to think and ask the question "Why?" or "Why not?"[1] is critical to stimulating their interest in research and to developing better ways to improve patient treatment within the confines of clinical practice. The plan is then simple: *demonstrate results, emphasize how research helped to obtain those results, and how research can be a positive determinant in better clinical responses.*

Does the Interest in Research Precede the Research Idea?

From my own perspective, interest in research comes first and then the research idea follows. However, it is possible that, in some cases, the research idea promotes the interest in research because of the necessity of solving the research idea. Both sequences are real. We need to be ready to approach the interest in research or the research idea, whichever comes first.

In subsequent chapters we will approach the best means to develop the research idea while here we concentrate on analyzing the importance of the interest in research. It is clear in the minds of many researchers that these various developments occur practically simultaneously. However, for academic purposes, it is critical that we separate the interest in research and the presence or evolution of the research idea.

The interest in research becomes an element that needs to be nourished through a series of examples, meetings, and defined research projects. The more the interest in research is applied, the more we can advance the cause of effective and consistent research. The interest in research is, above all, the pillar on which the research edifice rests.

References

[1] Hakim HS. Principles of Research. *Exper Clin Transpl.* 2007; 2-631-532.

[2] Booth WC, Colomb GG, Williams JM. *The Craft of Research.* The University of Chicago Press, Chicago, 1995.

[3] Toledo-Pereyra LH, *Passion for Surgical Research in* Toledo-Pereyra LH. (ed), *Vignettes on Surgery, History and Humanities.* Landes Bioscience, Georgetown, Texas, 2005.

[4] Toledo-Pereyra LH. *The Ethics of Surgical Research in* Toledo-Pereyra LH. (ed), *Vignettes on Surgery, History and Humanities.* Landes Bioscience, Georgetown, Texas, 2005.

[5] Toledo-Pereyra LH. Innovation in Toledo-Pereyra LH. (ed), *Innovation and Discovery on Surgery, History and Humanities.* Landes Bioscience, Austin, Texas, 2009.

In: Principles of Research
Editor: Luis H. Toledo-Pereyra
ISBN: 978-1-62417-968-6

Chapter 3

EVIDENCE-BASED MEDICINE

Luis H. Toledo-Pereyra
Western Michigan University School of Medicine,
Michigan State University College of Human Medicine,
Michigan State University College of Osteopathic Medicine,
Kalamazoo, MI, US

The good practice of medicine or surgery is dependent on the use of well-established research methods and recognized proven techniques, preferably derived from randomized clinical studies or systematic analyses. This is what we call today Evidence-Based Medicine or Evidence-Based Surgery.

Medicine or surgery, like many other disciplines have evolved by building personal experience upon personal experience. The knowledge initially was anecdotal and established through individual cases. Observation represented the most valuable ally under these conditions, and new advances were incorporated with a clear vision of modifying the patho-physiology encountered. Examples of this evolving system included many of the medical and surgical procedures we know today, such as diagnosis of diabetes mellitus, diagnosis and management of anemia, diagnosis and treatment of pneumonia, osteoporosis, urinary tract infections as well as hernia repair, appendectomy, small bowel obstruction treatment, cancer surgery, organ transplantation, and cardiac surgery. Good management of these diseases results and did not necessarily come from the system that we now call evidence-based medicine or surgery. How did this happen then? Is it possible that evidence-based medicine is just a new name for the same system we have always utilized? Can we continue practicing medicine as we have always done with good results and not mention evidence-based medicine? Let's see what explanation we use.

For fourteen years (1999-2013), while teaching the 18-hour annual course called *"Critical Analysis/Analytical Medicine"* (based entirely on the teachings of evidence-based medicine as proposed by Sackett and his group [1]) at Michigan State University College of Human Medicine in Kalamazoo, I initially thought that evidence-based medicine was not a new system. Indeed, I believed it to be the same system utilized since the ancient times of Hippocrates and the Greek natural school of medicine, continued by the great physicians Galen, Avicenna, Harvey, and many others into our present era. I could not believe, much less understand, how we had been practicing medicine and surgery for thousands of years – before evidence-based medicine debuted in 1992 [1-3] – incorporating progress, innovative knowledge, and new ways of treatment, supposedly without using evidence-based medicine and surgery. To me, this created an incongruity that was difficult to accept!

At this point, I went back to my surgical residency at the University of Minnesota (1970-1976) where I felt that science and research were at the forefront of our surgical activities, though without the name of evidence-based surgery. Other institutions of higher learning also had similar approaches to surgery without using the specific description of evidence-based medicine or surgery. Years after the term was coined in1992, physicians continued to make incredible discoveries based on a traditional understanding of science, research, and clinical experience. Where was evidence-based medicine then? And is it needed now?

It was not until I began being exposed to my teaching, *"Critical Appraisals/Analytical Medicine"* on the sixth year (2005) that I started to understand the enormous value that evidence-based medicine or surgery could provide. I guess it took me five years of study and teaching to better understand this approach to education. This special system's roots finally revealed its potential to me! I am a complete believer now and let me tell you why. Evidence-based medicine brought with it the application of systematic research to the traditional practice of medicine. It elevated the means by which a physician or surgeon, an evidence-based physician or surgeon, practice medicine or surgery and interpret and evaluate the literature to apply it ideally, that is with the understanding that statistics and study design enter into the final assessment of the patient or study results. According to evidence-based principles, the physician or surgeon should always ask three questions: Are the results valid? What are the results? And Are the results applicable to my patient? [1-12].

If David Sackett, distinguished clinician working until recently at McMaster University in Hamilton, Ontario, is considered the father of evidence-based medicine, certainly Archie Cochrane (1909-1988), noted British epidemiologist, should be considered the grandfather of this exciting medical movement. Cochrane was a dedicated proponent of randomized clinical trials, because he believed in their ability to provide the best clinical evidence when no one else was much interested. In 1972, he published his monumental work, *Effectiveness and Efficiency: Random Reflections on Health Services* [13, 14]. In it, he strongly supported the utilization of randomized trials to improve results and to test interventions. Even though the first randomized clinical trials came out in 1948 testing the role of streptomycin in treating tuberculosis, clinical epidemiology using randomized trials did not take hold until after Cochrane's book was published in 1972 [13-16]. In recognition of Cochrane's pioneering contributions to evidence-based medicine, Oxford University opened the first Cochrane Center in 1992, and a year later began the Cochrane Collaboration with other centers around the world [17-19].

Cochrane set the stage for Sackett and his group, who helped the surgical disciplines to accept evidence-based medicine as the basis for treatment and practice. Surgeons, encouraged by Cochrane's and Sackett's principles, addressed many key questions: How can we apply evidence-based medicine in a practical manner? What process allows us to implement evidence-based medicine effectively? What is evidence-based surgery? How can we qualify the evidence? How can we categorize the recommendations?

A definition of evidence-based medicine is extremely important, and it has already been presented at the beginning of this chapter. Let us add the definition given by the Centre for Evidence-Based Medicine: "Evidence-based medicine is the conscientious, explicit, and judicious use of current best evidence in making decisions about the care of individual patients" [20, 21]. The surgical ideal is making the best surgical decisions possible based on the gathering of the best evidence currently available. In order to reach this ideal, physicians and/or surgeons must access the literature that provides them with relevant information.

- First, identify the topic.
- Second, go to Pubmed/Medline
- Third, proceed to Cochrane database and systematic reviews
- Fourth, advance to *e-Medicine* and other well-known databases

These steps facilitate an exhaustive review that permits you to ascertain, without a doubt, the real and current status of the medical literature. The most updated and extensive database is Pubmed/Medline. The most carefully evaluated database for evidence-based medicine is the Cochrane database.

In order to characterize the type of evidence, we need to stratify the evidence qualitatively. In this regard, the U.S. Preventative Services Task Force has delineated five levels of evidence by defining the studies from which the clinical data emanated [10]. Level I is the highest evidence obtained from at least one randomized controlled trial. Level II-1 is the next in importance, with evidence gathered from a well-designed controlled trial without randomization; level II-2 is evidence obtained from well-designed cohort or case-control studies, preferable from several centers; level II-3 is evidence accumulated from multiple time series with our without intervention. Finally, level III, very anecdotal, is based in opinions of respected authorities, clinical experience, or reports of expert committees. This grading system, as good as it is, is not perfect since the relevance of measurements, the results of the study, and the baseline risk of the effect are not always included [10].

Another concern is the categorization of recommendations based on the level of evidence. The U.S. Preventative Service Task Force has defined three levels: level A, where the recommendations are based on good an consistent scientific evidence; level B, where the recommendations are based on limited or inconsistent scientific evidence; and level C, where the recommendations are based primarily on consensus and expert opinion n[10]. With this information, we can effectively categorize the level of evidence with the appropriate recommendations by strictly relying on the findings.

Robin McLeon presented an excellent review of evidence-based surgery from the surgeon's view-point in particular [9]. She discussed all elements of evidence-based medicine and surgery and reviewed issues of increasing importance for the practicing surgeon [9]. Issues of special concern for surgical trials were the standardization of the procedure and the surgeon's experience and ability to do the surgery. All aspects of perioperative and postoperative care should be standardized as well. One more point would be the performance of blind studies or sham operations which would be ethically difficult to justify in surgical trials today. Surgeons, then, should be aware of all of the various details in the practice of evidence-based surgery [22-29].

Before concluding, I should mention some statistics pertaining to evidence-based medicine. Around 9,000 randomized controlled trails and over two million articles in 10,000 medical journals are published every year [30]. This reflects the incredible and difficult task facing practicing physicians and surgeons who wish to keep up with this continuous and ever-increasing body of evidence. For example, an internist would have to read approximately 19 articles each day to stay current [30]. General surgeons would probably be required to review a similar number of papers daily to remain well informed. The impossibility of carrying out this awesome task requires that many medical or surgical decisions today be based frequently on personal expertise, the weakest form of evidence. In spite of the constraints and limitations of today's busy clinical work, future physicians and surgeons must learn to efficiently practice evidence-based medicine or surgery so that they can use the strongest form of evidence, the evidence based on scientific findings and well-established clinical trials.

How can evidence-based medicine or surgery be taught at the highest level of efficiency without seriously curtailing the physician or surgeon's current activities? I believe it can be done by incorporating the principles of evidence-based medicine into physicians or surgeons' daily rounds, operating room functions, postoperative treatment, and office practice. Only by integrating evidence-based principles into practice can we make our task simpler and the results worthwhile. When everyone practices evidence-based medicine or surgery, our ultimate objective of better patient care will be fully accomplished. We are looking forward to this day in the not too distant future.

REFERENCES

[1] Sackett Dl, Richardson WS, Rosenberg W, Haynes RB. *Evidence-Based Medicine: How To Practice 7 Teach EBM.* Edinburgh: Churchill Livingstone; 1998.

[2] Sacket DL, Richardson WS, Rosenberg W, Haynes RB. *How To Practice and Teach EBM*. New York: Churchill Livingstone; 1997.

[3] Sackett DL, Rosenberg WMC, Muir Gray, JA, Haynes RB, Richardson WS. Evidence based medicine: what it is and what it isn't. *BMJ*. 1996; 312:71-72. Available at: *http://bmj.bmjjournals.com/cgi/content/full/312/7023/71?eaf%2523r2*. Accessed August 1, 2005.

[4] Straus SE, Richardson WS, Glasziou P, Haynes RB. *Evidence-Based Medicine: How to Practice and Teach EBM*. Edinburgh: Elsevier Churchill Livingstone; 2005.

[5] Muir Gray JA. *Evidence-Based Healthcare: How To Make Health Policy and Management Decisions*. Edinburgh: Churchill Livingstone; 2001.

[6] Siwek J, Gourlay ML, Slawson DC, Shaughnessy AF. How to write an evidence-based clinical review article. *Am Fam Physician*. 2002; 65(2). Available at: http://www.aafp.org/afp/2002115/251.html. Accessed August 1, 2005.

[7] Olkin I. Statistical and theoretical considerations in metaanalysis. *J Clin Epidemiol.* 1995;48:133-146.

[8] Ellis J, Mulligan I, Rowe J, Sackett DL. Inpatient general medicine is evidence based. *Lancet*. 1995;346:407-110.

[9] McLeod RS. Evidence-based surgery. In: Norton JA et al, eds. *Surgery: Basic Science and Clinical Evidence*. New York: Springer-Verlag; 2001.

[10] Evidence-Based Medicine. Available at: *http://en.wikipedia.org/wiki/ Evidence-based_medicine*. Accepted August 1, 2005.

[11] Barton S. Using clinical evidence. *BMJ.* 2001;322-503-504. Available at: *http://bmj.bmjjournals.com/cgi/content/full/322/7285/503*. Accessed August 1, 2005.

[12] Urschel JD, Goldsmith CH, Tandan VR, Miller JD. Users' guide to evidence-based surgery: how to use an article evaluating surgical interventions. *An J Surg* 2001;44:95-100.

[13] Culp K. History: Archie Cochrane. Available at: *http://www.smj. org.uk/0802/cochrane.htm*. Accessed August 3, 2005.

[14] Hill GB. Archie Cochrane and his legacy. An internal challenge to physicians' autonomy? *J Clin Epidemiol.* 2000; 53(12);1189-1192.

[15] Alvarez-Dardet C, Ruiz MT. Thomas McKeown and Archibald Cochrane: a journey through the diffusion of their ideas. *BMJ.* 1993;306(6887):1252-1254.

[16] Archie Cochrane-Publications. Available at: *http://www.cardiff.ac.uk/ schoolsand divisions/divisions/insrv/libraryservices/ research/cochrane.* Accessed August 3, 2005.

[17] Alvarao Nagib A. The Cochrane collaboration in the third world. *Sao Palo Med J*. 1998; 116(3). Available at: *http://www.scielo.br/scielo.php? script=sci_arttext&pid=S1516-31801998000300001*. Accessed August 3, 2005.

[18] Archie Cochrane Archive-Cardiff University. Available at: *http://www.cardiff.ac.uk/schoolsanddivisions/divisions/insrv/libraryservices/research/cochrane*. Accessed August 3, 2005.

[19] The name behind the 'Cochrane' Collaboration. Available at: http://www.cochrane.org/docs/archieco.htm. Accessed August 2, 3005.

[20] Scalise D. Evidence-based medicine. *Hospitals & Health Networks*. December 15, 2004. Available at: *http://www.hhnmag.com/hhnmag/*

hospitalconnect/search/articl.jsp?dcrpath=HHNMAG. Accessed August 1, 2005.

[21] Center for Health Evidence. *Evidence-Based Medicine: A New Approach to Teaching and the Practice of Medicine*. Available at: *http://www. cche.net/usersguides/ebm.asp*. Accessed August 15, 2005.

[22] Wente MN, Seiler CM, Uhl W, Buchler MW. Perspectives of evidence-based surgery. *Dig Surg*. 2003;20(4):263-269.

[23] Black N. Evidence-based surgery: A passing fad? *World J Surg*. 1999;23(8):789-793.

[24] Saurland S. Lefering R, Neugebauer EAM. The pros and cons of evidence-based surgery. *Langenbeck's Arch Surg*. 1999;384(5):423-431.

[25] Stirrat GM. Ethics and evidence based surgery. *J Med Ethics*. 2004;30:160-165.

[26] Gentileschi P, Kini S, Catarci M, Gagner M. Evidence-based medicine: open and laparoscopic bariatric surgery. *Surgical Endoscopy*. 2002;16(5):736-744.

[27] Baraldini V, Spitz L, Pierro A. Evidence-based operations in pediatric surgery. *Pediatr Surg Int*. 1998;13:331-335.

[28] Searching for the Best Evidence in Clinical Journals. Available at: *http://www.cebm.net/searching.asp*. Assessed August 1, 2005.

[29] Gordon T, Cameron J, eds. *Evidence-Based Surgery*. B.C. Decker; 2000.

[30] Antes G, Falck-Ytter Y, and trautmann N. Evidence-Based Medicine and the Cochrane Collaboration. Available at: *www. goinginternational.org/english/pdf/archive/Antes_ua_e.pdf*. Accessed August 15, 2005.

In: Principles of Research
Editor: Luis H. Toledo-Pereyra

ISBN: 978-1-62417-968-6

Chapter 4

RESEARCH IDEA

Luis H. Toledo-Pereyra
Western Michigan University School of Medicine,
Michigan State University College of Human Medicine,
Michigan State University College of Osteopathic Medicine,
Kalamazoo, MI, US

INTRODUCTION TO THE RESEARCH IDEA

After the interest in research, developing the research idea is of fundamental importance because without it we cannot have research. Where do the research ideas come from then? Is there any better way to improve our ability to generate research ideas? Where do they come from? What are the factors that stimulate the research idea?

Anything we do in and out of medicine or surgery should be the force that will maintain our mind occupied on our future research ideas. From events in the clinical arena to discussions in formal rounds or informal meetings should be the origin of our thinking in research. So, the generations of research ideas come from any place and we should be aware of it. We could be successful in research if we could produce and accumulate the ideas as they frequently present to us in our professional or daily life. The research environment could help us in securing the presence and evolution of the idea. Be aware of changes and future developments and be ready to admit and grow the research idea that could be presented to you during the practice of medicine.

The research idea usually comes from interest, knowledge and desire to obtain an appropriate answer regarding the problem identified. Asking specific questions about the areas of interest will be very helpful in defining the research idea.

The research idea is not difficult to develop when you use an inquisitive mind and attitude towards finding responses to the questions presented. The research idea would then offer a guiding light to the research process.

SOURCES FOR THE RESEARCH IDEA

For the researcher, the research idea comes naturally and is immediately incorporated into a good research protocol. The difficulty might arise for those individuals who are unfamiliar with research, and thus the research idea does not readily present itself. These individuals need support to reach an appropriate research idea. It is possible that at this stage the most effective manner to reach the research idea is by examining the most diverse possibilities and questions in the areas of concern. Then the next step would be to select the best idea.

The research idea is important because the results of the project are dependent on its elaboration and execution based on a well-outlined research plan. Good research ideas are the basis for the development of excellent protocols and, at the same time, for the integration of successful studies with the best conclusions.

The research idea proceeds from many sources, such as a literature review, reference books, specialty books on the topic in question, analysis of the discussions emanating from floor rounds, Grand Rounds and other internal conferences utilized by the various teaching residency programs. Members of the faculty will frequently present interesting points which medical students, residents and faculty could utilize as potential sources for excellent research ideas and potential review or full analysis of the topic under consideration.

EVOLUTION OF THE RESEARCH IDEA

The research idea represents the first exposure of the researcher or the researcher-to-e to the possibility of advancing the first steps of the research project. The research idea can be heterogeneous, multifaceted, and only limited by the imaginative capability of the investigator. The research idea, of course, can be very simple and clearly visible from the beginning. The research idea can be present in any possible form.

The research idea responds to the "whys" of a clinical case, a particular situation or problem that presents in daily practice and can be very satisfying when appropriately addressed. Nadey Hakim, well-known English transplant surgeon, put it very clearly when discussing the research idea [1]. He wrote, "The research idea must be original. It could be an observation; it could come from talks, lectures…or it could be personal inquisitiveness and dreaming"[1]. Hakim continued his discussion by invoking science philosopher Karl Popper, who said, "What a good teacher says is this: Try to learn what people are discussing nowadays in science. Find out where difficulties arise and take interest in disagreement. These are the questions you should take up" [2].

As suggested before by Popper, researchers should not be afraid to approach difficult issues or questions arising from controversial topics [2]. On the contrary, researchers searching for research ideas should be aware that research ideas can originate from unsettled or unsolved clinical issues. It would not be hard to understand, then, that difficult topics or challenging areas are excellent sources for research ideas [3].

FACTORS THAT STIMULATE THE RESEARCH IDEA

As previously mentioned, the research idea is frequently stimulated by thoughts that the clinicians have while performing their usual duties. The research idea can frequently center around clinical concerns and the ability to solve these issues effectively. Let's present for a brief moment a surgical and medical case as an example of a potential research idea.

In surgery, we could examine the best characterized issues, such as preoperative assessment, details of the operation and its performance, modification of the surgical technique, postoperative follow-up, and final results, including morbidity and mortality. The research idea could come from more specific topics related to the previous general topics. One could approach, for instance, the differences and outcomes of laparoscopic inguinal hernioplasty vs. regular open hernia repair. Other ideas could be oriented toward the proper surgical procedure, such as which suture is best. What is the best tissue approximation? How many layers should be sutured? Many more research questions could follow, covering a large number of simple or intricate areas worth exploring in better understanding of hernia disease and/or treatment.

In medicine, the origin, diagnosis and treatment of the disease take precedence over strictly surgical matters. If we follow, for example, the topic of hypertensive disease, there are many research ideas that could emerge from careful consideration of the disease course. Simple or complex research ideas could appear, stimulated by the desire to have more precise diagnosis and/or treatment. An example could be to define ideal blood pressure levels, or the most important contributing factors for improved survival, or the best treatment of maintaining optimal blood pressure measurements. These are just a few examples of the many research ideas that could be entertained in the clinical arena. Literature review topics can also be a rich source of many promising research ideas. The research idea development becomes, at this point, so extensive that the possibilities for study are practically inexhaustible.

Conclusion

It is well-known in the realm of the clinical or basic sciences that the development of the research idea is the central element in the creation of a significant research protocol, and, thereafter, a good experimental design and the institution of a complete research study. Stimulating the sources of the research idea and knowing the factors that could potentially enhance better ideas is fundamental to improving the research process. The research idea is the critical step needed for research advancement in the medical and surgical sciences.

References

[1] Hakim NS. Principles of research. *Exper Clin Transpl.* 2007;2,631-632.

[2] Popper K. *Conjectures and Refutations. The Growth of Scientific Knowledge.* 5th Ed. Oxford Univ. Press, United Kingdom, 2002.

[3] Toledo-Pereyra LH. Importance of medical and surgical research. *J. Invest Surg.* 2009;22:325-326.

In: Principles of Research
Editor: Luis H. Toledo-Pereyra
ISBN: 978-1-62417-968-6

Chapter 5

RESEARCH HYPOTHESIS

Luis H. Toledo-Pereyra[1], Benedict Dormitorio[2], Alexander H. Toledo[3] and Robert Flikkema[2]

[1]Western Michigan University School of Medicine,
Michigan State University College of Human Medicine,
Michigan State University College of Osteopathic Medicine,
Kalamazoo, MI, US
[2]Western Michigan University, Department of Statistics,
Kalamazoo, Michigan, US
[3]University of North Carolina,
Division of Abdominal Organ Transplantation, Chapel Hill, NC, US

INTRODUCTION TO THE RESEARCH HYPOTHESIS

The research hypothesis is fundamental to the completion of the research study. The research hypothesis is needed for a sound and well-developed research study. The research hypothesis contributes to the solution of the research problem. Without the research hypothesis, we cannot learn all the critical elements of the research process and the conclusions would be limited in their reach [1-11].

The elaboration of a research hypothesis permits a better definition of the statistical method to be considered for the study in question. A good research hypothesis helps to further clarify details of the statistical method. Finally, a good research hypothesis helps to understand the statistical framework within the context of the whole project.

In this chapter we analyze two aspects of the research hypothesis, one related to the characterization of the research hypothesis, and another one pertaining to the formulation and basis for a well-defined hypothesis.

IMPORTANCE OF THE RESEARCH HYPOTHESIS

The research hypothesis is the basis upon which the research project is built and that is of particular importance to the overall success of the protocol. Having a well-planned hypothesis will help to secure the completion of a good protocol [8].

Now, how do you ensure that the hypothesis is clearly presented? Is there a way to frequently reach this significant possibility? I believe we can reach this stage by being aware of the elements included in a good hypothesis, elements such as the development of an acceptable question based on a reasonable and logical problem, and a complete review of the literature as well.

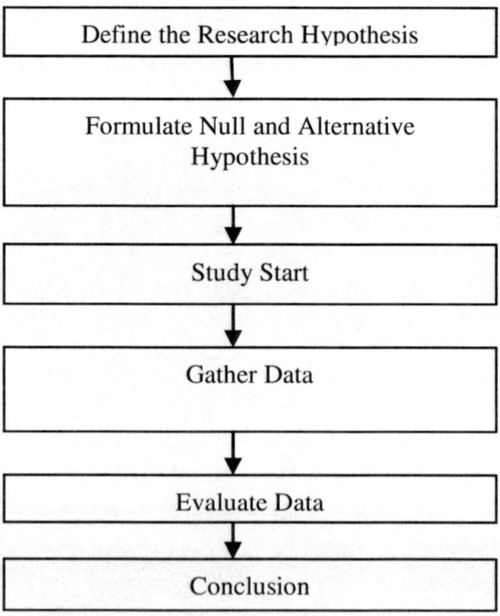

Figure 1. Hypothesis statistical testing from defining the research hypothesis to evaluating the data and conclusion.

The importance of the research hypothesis is directly dependent on previously known facts, potential solutions, and expected results from the variables analyzed. The hypothesis is then at the center of the research study, the research data obtained, and the conclusions reached. With the data collected and carefully reviewed, the hypothesis can be supported or not based on the findings that have been gathered. In brief, the hypothesis is essential to the research study [9].

Definition of the Research Hypothesis

A research hypothesis has many faces, but a good definition should include phrases such as "stating the research problem", "characterizing the questions posed in the protocol", and "defining the conclusions reached". A research hypothesis is clear, well-defined, and covers the essential basis of the problem. To have a good hypothesis is to have the important ingredients for the completion of a good study.

The scope of a research hypothesis should be supported by the findings of the protocol. The hypothesis according to Gay and Associates [3] "*is a refinement of the research problem.*" Supporting and/or testing the research hypothesis with reliable data represent the best means to make the study worthwhile.

Formulating the Research Hypothesis

To formulate the research hypothesis can be very simple, depending on the protocol undertaken, or very complex if the study has many variables that need close correlation and full assessment of their value.

The formulation of the problem precedes the formulation of the hypothesis. However, the literature review precedes both of them, since knowledge of the literature will facilitate the understanding of the principles or findings to be corroborated or challenged.

The ability to test the hypothesis is fundamental to proving that the elements of it are right or wrong. Testability of the hypothesis is critical to defining its validity. When formulating the hypothesis, the logic should be clear and organized to readily demonstrate its strength.

The hypothesis is formulated when we have enough information to determine if the problem or variables sought can be tested and compared to each other. Hypothesis testing is needed in the majority of research studies, except those that remain exploratory or have not been well-defined yet. In this way, the hypothesis should be formulated at the right time and with the right set of variables. Thus, the problem is first presented, the literature reviewed next, and the hypothesis formulated thereafter (Figures 1, 2).

TYPES OF RESEARCH HYPOTHESIS

There are several types of research hypotheses, such as the inductive (based on observation) or deductive (originating from theory), the directional (expected direction) or non-directional (relation exists), and the null (no significant relation) and alternative (significant relation) hypotheses [2].

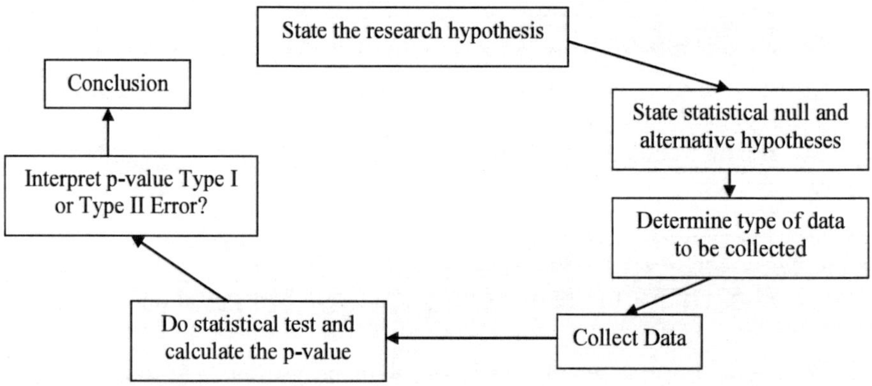

Figure 2. Hypothesis development from beginning to end.

From the statistical point of view, the null and alternative hypotheses are used. The null hypothesis predicts no significant difference, which is shown as H_o. The alternative hypothesis demonstrates a significant difference, which is characterized by H_A or H_1 [5].

The null hypothesis originates from a probability that cannot be demonstrated to be true. The alternative hypothesis originates from unbiased analysis of the rejection of the null hypothesis, resulting in acceptance of the alternative hypothesis. These goals are always pursued for statistically significant research (Figure 2).

Conclusion

As indicated in figure 2, hypothesis development include the determination of the null and alternative hypotheses, collection of the data and evaluation of it, with interpretation of the p-value as to whether type I or type II error are to be considered and a final conclusion reached. These steps already well-represented in figure 2 are the cornerstone of hypothesis development and testing.

References

[1] Bartoszynski R, Niewiadomska-Bugaj M. *Probability Statistical Inference*. 2nd ed. Wiley-Interscience; 2008.

[2] Browner WS, Newman TB, Cummings SR, Hully SB. Getting Ready to Estimate Sample Size: Hypotheses and Underlying Principles. In Hully SB and Cummings SR. *Designing Clinical Research.* Williams and Wilkins; 1988:128-138.

[3] Gay L, Mills G, Airasian P. *Educational research; Competencies for Analysis and Application. 8th Ed.* Upper Saddle River, NJ: Prentice-Hall; 2006.

[4] Hakim NS. Principles of Research. *Exp Clin. Transpl.* 2007;5:631-632.

[5] Sheskin DJ. *Handbook of Parametric and Nonparametric Statistical Procedures.* 2nd ed. Boca Raton, Florida: Chapman & Hall/CRC; 2000.

[6] Souba WW, Wilmore DW, eds. *Surgical Research.* San Diego, California: Academic Press; 1991.

[7] Toledo-Pereyra LH. Becoming a Surgical Scholar. *J Invest Surg*. 2011; 24:139-140.

[8] Toledo-Pereyra LH. Developing the Research Idea. *J Invest Surg*. 2011; 24:101-102.

[9] Toledo-Pereyra LH. Interest in Surgical Research. *J Invest Surg*. 2011; 24:99-100.

[10] Utts JM, Heckard RF. *Mind on Statistics*. 3rd ed. Belmont, California: Thomson Brooks/Cole; 2007.

[11] Toledo AH, Flikkema R, Toledo-Pereyra LH. Developing the Research Hypothesis. *J. Invest Surg*. 2011; 24:191-194.

In: Principles of Research
Editor: Luis H. Toledo-Pereyra

ISBN: 978-1-62417-968-6

Chapter 6

RESEARCH DESIGN

Luis H. Toledo-Pereyra
Western Michigan University School of Medicine,
Michigan State University College of Human Medicine,
Michigan State University College of Osteopathic Medicine,
Kalamazoo, MI, US

INTRODUCTION

The development of a good research design permits us to obtain the best research data possible. From the experimental question to the research hypothesis and data collection of variables we can begin to consider the optimal research design. Details pertaining to the selection of the research design are considered within and very much in relation with the knowledge of the researcher and the support of his research group.

The research design represents the first step in organizing and planning the research process once the research idea and research hypothesis have been clearly outlined. In regard to the research design, we need to establish the best research plan to obtain the most accurate results possible. The study of the research knowledge reached by other investigators orients us to decipher the research question in the most critical manner. The research design would have to be clear, appropriately conceived and based on logical concepts to advance in the best possible way the research concept being developed.

DESIGNING THE STUDY

It is not that simple to ascertain the best design available for the research study in question. Some variables or considerations will be different depending on whether the study is experimental (eg. animals) or clinical (eg. humans) since experimental studies are more dependent on the experimental model and the availability of tests to define the question(s) under consideration. For the clinical study the planning extends into whether the study should be retrospective, prospective or on occasion a combination of the two done at different times. The clinical study considers more frequently the possibility of randomization and the extended variables associated with it. The clinical study needs to control all clinical parameters which frequently are more difficult to restrict and/or eliminate than in the experimental study.

In establishing a good research design, whether clinical or experimental, we need to focus on the research question and equally important on the research hypothesis as well [1-4]. That is the research design should allow the researcher to gather measurements and information about the variables in consideration from the least amount of subjects or experimental units as well as taking minimal time and other resources. When the research question and hypothesis are clear and well-defined, the research design becomes more evident and readily introduced in the overall planning of the study.

Let us present two examples as a way to explain the design associated with various types of research [5, 6]. On the one hand we can consider an experimental study dealing, for example, with the role of allopurinol in mice or rats undergoing liver ischemia. Knowing that the model of liver ischemia is well-accepted and has been previously studied and that the end-points are clearly defined, we can then study the precise dose and timing of administration of allopurinol regarding its protective effect in ischemic liver tissue [5]. Details of other questions to be presented and analyzed in subsequent experiments should be considered under the conditions of new experiments. The use of several other drugs, the interaction of the various parameters being studied, the advancement of the ischemia field pertaining to better results and the improved understanding of the mechanisms of organ and cell damage are just some of the possibilities to be considered when planning new or previously undefined experiments.

On the other hand, we have the clinical setting of experiments and how to plan them well so that we can use good questions, advanced hypotheses and improved means to recognize the best parameters to analyze in the clinical study to be designed. In this case, let us assume we have a clinical study that is investigating whether patients with coronary heart disease can show clinical improvement when treated with allopurinol, an old drug used for the treatment of gout and now considered as an anti-ischemic medication [5, 6]. How to plan or design these experiments when studying this group of patients remains an important question. Needless to say, the best study will be a randomized prospective trial where we utilize good parameters of ischemic injury and set up acceptable goals to reach under these conditions.

We would need then to define the dose and timing of the administration of allopurinol. A good literature search will offer the best source to define the optimal dose used so far in situations like the one presented [5, 6]. Regarding the research design, an optimal control group is essential because of the necessity of having the best comparative base against which the treated group will be analyzed. Acceptable parameters for assessing ischemic injury will be utilized and randomization for control and treatment groups will be introduced. Within the planning phase, the number of patients to treat will be defined as will be the statistical analysis to be used.

With the experiment in process, collection of data on the parameters agreed upon will be essential in order to have the appropriate information that reflects the effect of allopurinol in coronary ischemic conditions [6]. Statistical analysis will follow and evaluation of the whole experiment will enter into place. Now, conclusions will be entertained and the researcher (s) will begin writing the evidence obtained.

TYPES OF RESEARCH STUDIES

Within the design of the research study, we can encounter many types of studies that need to be accepted or eliminated according to the protocol being examined. In this regard, one good way to divide the research design is in 3 types: 1. randomized experiment when randomization was used; 2. quasi-experimental design when randomization was not used but multiple groups or several measurements were undertaken; and 3. non-experimental design when no randomization or multiple groups or measurements were utilized. It is obvious that number 1 will be the best design to evaluate internal validity or causal assessment [1-4]. However, the best decision will depend on the research question, the hypothesis examined and the goals of the researcher pertaining to the groups needed or parameters to be utilized in the study being carried out.

When designing a new study, is important to keep in mind that research studies can also be descriptive (incidence of outcomes over time), analytic (evaluation of risk factors associated to outcomes), prospective (variables studied before outcomes occur) and retrospective (variables studied after outcomes have occurred [4].

Within the elaboration of the research design, the use of cohort studies (group of patients followed over time) is worth considering as well since utilizing the cohort concept completes thoroughly the study of the data. Adding this element into the research allows the researchers to study risk factors with respect to time (eg. is drug A more effective in the early phase of the treatment compared to a later time point?). The cohort study can either be a prospective cohort study or a retrospective cohort study. Both of them have strengths and weaknesses based on the inherent selection of patients and variables associated with the study [4]. Furthermore, sometimes it may be necessary to add a double-cohort study, used more frequently in occupational and environmental medicine where different exposures are presented to a potential risk factor and outcome differences are the basis for evaluating the final results [4].

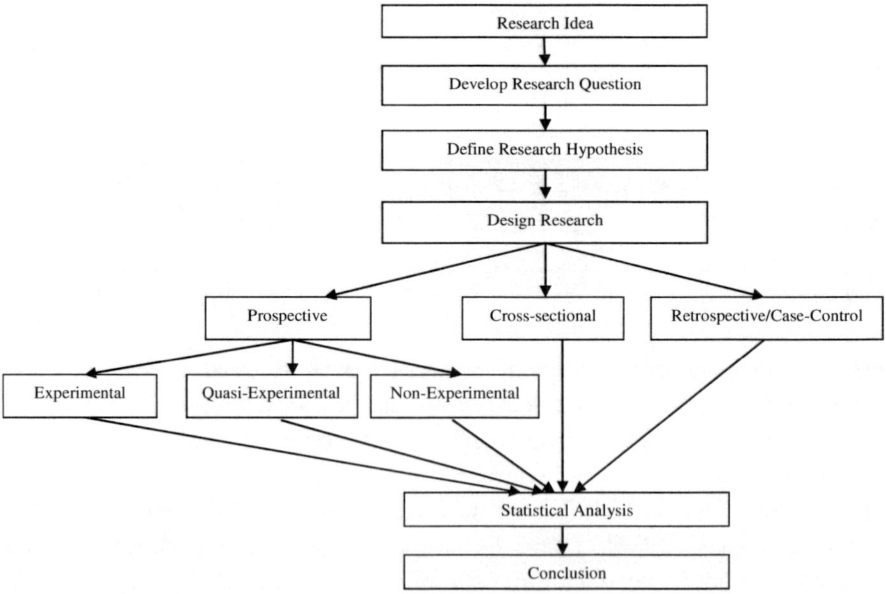

Figure 1. Research design relative to the study.

Careful attention needs to be placed on the presence of confounding variables since they can alter the results of the research study. These variables are associated with the predictor (factors being studied) and the outcome data [4]. For prospective studies, the effect of the confounding variable can be eliminated or minimized buy allocating the grouping (eg. treatment versus placebo) evenly on the values of the confounding variables. The confounding variables need to be defined early in the development of the study to prevent misconception of results.

When designing a new study, cross-sectional and case-control studies need to be characterized in the study planning period. In the cross-sectional research study, all measurements are made on one occasion. In the case-control study, the prevalence of risk factors in patients with a disease is compared to those patients without the disease [1-4].

Finally, a randomized blinded trial has been considered as the optimal trial in assessing the results obtained from a well-defined research study. Hulley and associates [4] have defined six steps in designing a carefully planned randomized blinded trial: 1. select a sample from the population, 2. measure baseline variables, 3. randomize subjects or otherwise, 4. apply interventions with a blinded placebo, 5. follow up the cohorts and, 6. measure outcome variables blindly if possible.

CONCLUSION

It is evident that the research design is essential in developing a good and worthwhile research study. From the conception of the idea and research hypothesis is necessary to define which ones are the critical elements to be included in the research design.

Considering the potential results we are theoretically seeking allow us to develop the best research design in question. Elements of various research designs have been introduced within this work.

REFERENCES

[1] Beveridge WIB. *The Art of Scientific Investigation*. Vintage Books, New York.1957.

[2] Creswell JW. *Research Design. Qualitative, Quantitative, and Mixed methods Approaches.* SAGE Publications. Thousand Oaks, CA, 2003.

[3] Rosas y Novelo ML. *La Ciencia y el Metodo Experimental.* UNAM, Mexico, 1990.

[4] *Hulley SB, Cummings SR. Designing* Clinical Research. Williams and Wilkins, Baltimore, 1998.

[5] Peglow S, Toledo AH, Anaya-Prado R, Lopez –Neblina F, Toledo-Pereyra LH. Allopurinol and Xanthine Oxidase Inhibition in Liveer Ischemia Reperfusion. *J Hepatobiliary Pancreat Sc*, 2011; 18:137-146.

[6] Lee BE, Toledo AH, Anaya-Prado R, Roach RR, Toledo-Pereyra LH. Allopurinol, Xanthine Oxidase and Cardiac Ischemia. *J Invest Med*, 2009; 57:902-909.

In: Principles of Research
Editor: Luis H. Toledo-Pereyra
ISBN: 978-1-62417-968-6

Chapter 7

STATISTICAL ANALYSIS

***Benedict Dormitorio*[1], *Robert Flikkema*[1], *Alexander H. Toledo*[2] *and Luis H. Toledo-Pereyra*[3]**

[1]Western Michigan University, Department of Statistics, Kalamazoo, MI, US

[2]University of North Carolina, Division of Abdominal Organ Transplantation, Chapel Hill, NC

[3]Western Michigan University School of Medicine, Michigan State University College of Human Medicine, Michigan State University College of Osteopathic Medicine, Kalamazoo, MI, US

INTRODUCTION TO STATISTICS

Statistics play a crucial role in any research analysis and development. Like any other scientific discipline, medicine requires a vigorous assessment of the data obtained. Statistics, the science of data analysis can thoroughly help to determine the real value of a medical or surgical intervention.

Statistical methods are an integral part of medical research. One cannot produce high quality medical or surgical research without considering the application of the most appropriate and accepted statistical procedures (1-13). Since statistical methods to be used in research depend on optimizing the information gathered, selection of an appropriate method becomes extremely important. To cover the most common problems in medical research, this chapter will discuss statistical methods designed to analyze numerical and categorical variables for two or more groups.

General Hypothesis Testing Procedures

Hypothesis testing is a set of statistical methods which aim to help the researcher to determine which of two possible conclusions the data support. For example, if a researcher would like to find out the effect of a new drug in reducing blood sugar levels on diabetic patients, he/she would have to weigh the data and point out which of the following two statements he/she supports; either the new drug reduces blood sugar or the new drug does not reduce blood sugar levels.

In this regard, the use of p-value becomes a fundamental part of the analysis. Briefly, p-value is the probability of observing the data when the null hypothesis is true. Following this definition, a small p-value indicates that the null hypothesis is not true. The same applies for a large p value that indicates that the null hypothesis is true. Typically, a hypothesis test is evaluated at 0.05 level of significance, which means that if a p value is below 0.05 then there is a small chance that the null hypothesis is true and therefore rejecting it.

Tests For Numerical Data Involving Two Groups

One of the most common problems in medical research is comparing two groups with respect to a numerical measure. For this problem, there are two common tests used to assess the differences between the two groups; the Mann-Whitney U test and the Two Sample t-test [10].

The type of test selected depends on the data. If it can be assumed that the data is drawn from a normally distributed population (bell shaped distribution), then, a Two Sample t-test is the appropriate test. On the other hand, the Mann-Whitney U test is considered a non-parametric test because it does not assume on the data being selected from a population of a particular distribution and therefore can be used with any sample data.

If one is unsure if normality of the population can be assumed, there are many normality tests that can be used. Some examples include the Shapiro-Wilks test, the D'Agostino k-squared test and the Anderson-Darling test [9].

EXAMPLE

Given below are the descriptive statistics for average age of two particular groups. The first group included people that were given the drug allopurinol in a study while the second group was a control group that was not given allopurinol [12]. The variable being investigated as the age of the two groups. Allopurinol is a xanthine oxidase inhibitor that reduces the amount of uric acid in the human body [7, 12]. The table below presents the results.

	Mean	Standard Deviation	Sample Size	*P*-value
Allopurinol Group	59.275	8.882	230	0.11
Control Group	60.912	12.427	209	

Assume that a normality test was run and the populations did not significantly differ from normality. The researcher would then decide to run a 2-Sample *t*-test to see if the means of 59.275 and 60.921 are significantly different. The two sided *P*-value of 0.11 implies that the means do not significantly differ between the two groups since it is greater than the significance level of 0.05.[1]

TESTS FOR NUMERICAL DATA INVOLVING MORE THAN TWO GROUPS

The parametric test for more than two groups is called analysis of variance (ANOVA). Like the 2-Sample *t*-test, ANOVA assumes that the samples are taken from a normally distributed population. ANOVA also assumes equal variances between all groups. If this assumption is not met, there are other tests such as the Welch test that can be used. ANOVA compares all the means of the different groups all at once and therefore maintains a 0.05 significance level.. However, there are limitations to ANOVA. The null hypothesis in an ANOVA test is "all the means are equivalent" while the alternative hypothesis is "all means are not equivalent". Rejection of the null hypothesis does not complete the analysis since ANOVA by itself does not tell us which of the sample means or how many of them are different. There might be only one mean that differs from the others or they could all be different from one another. That's why a significant ANOVA *P*-value needs to be followed by a post-hoc analysis using one of several different methods including the Bonferroni, Tukey and Dunnett tests [2].

The Kruskal-Wallis test is similar to the Mann-Whitney U test since it is based on the ranks of the data and therefore can be used with data selected from any distribution. The Kruskal-Wallis test suffers from the same problem as ANOVA does with its hypotheses. A significant Kruskal-Wallis *P*-value needs to be followed by appropriate post-hoc analysis. The Bonferonni test is valid for non-parametric data in addition to parametric data and can be used.

The following study investigated four groups and their anastomic bursting pressure. The question of interest is for which groups the bursting pressure differs.

EXAMPLE

	Anastomic bursting pressure (mm HG)	Standard Deviation
Group 1	81.1	23.83
Group 2	32.33	26.06
Group 3	15.87	11.36
Group 4	17.62	18.02

The appropriate procedure is ANOVA since there are more than two groups. The ANOVA *P*-value is <0.05; this indicates that not all the means are the same. However, ANOVA does not tell us which specific groups are different and which are the same. In order to determine this, Tukey tests need to be implemented.

Group compared	Tukey p-value
1 vs. 2	0.003
1 vs. 3	0.0001
1 vs. 4	0.0001
2 vs. 3	0.05
2 vs. 4	0.05
3 vs. 4	0.05

Based on the Tukey *P*-values, it can be seen that Group 1 significantly differs from the other three groups. However, none of the Group 2, 3, or 4 comparisons indicate significantly different means.

About Categorical Data

Categorical or discrete data (variables that can only assume fixed values; eg. Gender) comes in two forms. The first is known as nominal data, which is composed of unordered categories. The second type is known as ordinal data, which is composed of ordered categories. The simplest form of categorical data analysis involves comparing two categories between two groups. This setup can be expanded to compare more than two categories between two groups and can go as far as comparing multiple categories between multiple groups.

The first test for analyzing categorical data is known as the Chi-Square test [8]. The Chi-Square test is one of the most well known and widely used statistical tests available since it can be used for categorical comparisons involving any number of categories. The null hypothesis for a Chi-Square is always that there is no treatment effect between groups while the alternative hypothesis is that there is some treatment effect. Similar to the ANOVA hypothesis test, a significant Chi-Square *P*-value can be followed up with a post-hoc analysis to determine what the treatment effect is.

In the following example we are testing to see if the proportion of people who took the anticoagulant warfarin differs between two groups.

Example

	Allopurinol Group	Control Group	P-value
Warfarin	10	8	0.564
No Warfarin	36	21	

The first group is a study group that was given allopurinol while the second group is a control group that was not given any medication. The first thing to notice is that every observation in our data set falls into one of four pre-determined categories. These categories are allopurinol and warfarin, allopurinol and no warfarin, control and warfarin, and control and no warfarin. All of our cells have over 5 observations so it would be reasonable to use a Chi-Square test. If one of our cells had a frequency less than 5, we would have to use Fisher's test.

The Chi-Square test produces a *P*-value of 0.564**. Since the *P*-value is greater than 0.05, the proportion of people who took warfarin does not significantly differ between the two groups.

General Overview of a Statistical Procedure

In the chart presented before, we can observe the general flow that an appropriate statistical test should follow. Once the surgical research study has been defined and the study design has been agreed upon, the data collection will be gathered and thereafter analyzed. The investigator in consultation with the statistician will decide what data is available, whether categorical or numerical. Based on the type of data, the test will be selected and a conclusion reached.

Flowchart of General Statistical Procedure

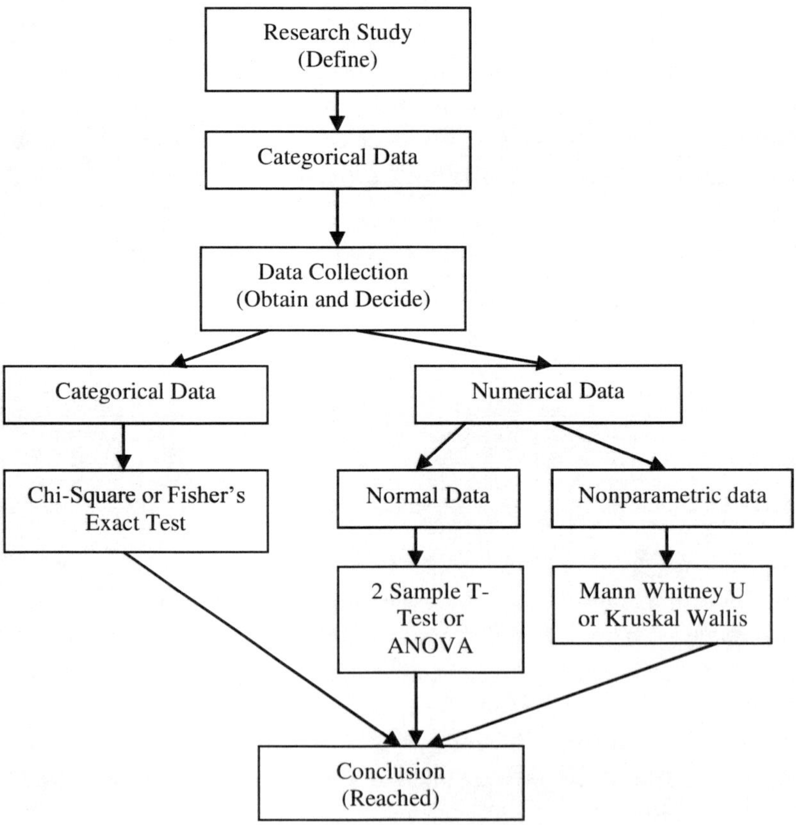

Conclusion

Statistics are of paramount importance in medical or surgical research since an inadequate sample size or an incorrect statistical procedure can undermine the entire study. Good statistics simplify the understanding and proper application of surgical research. In this way, a researcher can obtain more uniform data. Important tests common to surgical research include the 2-Sample *t*-test, the Mann-Whitney U test, Kruskal-Wallis, ANOVA, Chi-Square test and Fisher's Exact test. Additionally the surgical researcher must consider the appropriate sample size to obtain medically significant results. The correct use of the aforementioned methods will lead to meaningful and valid medical or surgical research.

References

[1] Bakoyannis G, Touloumi G. Practical methods for competing risks data: A review. *Statistical Methods in Medical Research*. Sevenoaks, Kent, UK, January 2011.

[2] Bartoszynski R, Niewiadomska-Bugaj M. *Probability Statistical Inference*. 2nd. Ed. Wiley-Interscience; 2008.

[3] Bhatia R, Wier M. 'Safety in Numbers' re-examined: can we make valid or practical inferences from available evidence? *Accident, Analysis and Prevention*. 2011; 34:235-40.

[4] Ceppi M, Gallo F, Bonassi S. Study design and statistical analysis of data in human population studies with the micronucleus assay. *Mutagenesis*. 2011; 26:247-52.

[5] Hu LP, Bao XL, Guan X. Statistical inference and experimental design of univariate qualitative data of single-group design (part one). *Journal of Chinese Integrative Medicine*. 2010; 8:888-92.

[6] Irkorucu O, Ucan B, Karadeniz G, et al. Effect of 2-OctylCyanoacrylate on Ischemic Anastomosis of the Left Colon. *Journal of Investigative Surgery*. 2009; 22:188-94.

[7] Netzloff C, Murty P, Lewis K, Gallardo GE, Toledo-Pereyra LH. Protective Effect of Allopurinol in Coronary Artery Disease: Phase II. *29th annual Kalamazoo Community Medical and Health Sciences Research Day Program Book*. Pp 24, April 2011.

[8] O'Leary JP. Ed. *The Physiologic Basis of Surgery.* 3rd ed. New Orleans, Louisiana: Lippincott Williams & Wilkins; 2002.

[9] Sheskin DJ. *Handbook of Parametric and Nonparametric Statistical Procedures.* 2nd ed. Boca Raton, Florida: Chapman & Hall/CRC;2000.

[10] Souba WW, Wilmore DW, eds. *Surgical Research.* San Diego, California: academic Press; 1991.

[11] Utts JM, Heckard RF. *Mind on Statistics.* 3rd ed. Belmont, California: Thomson Brooks/Cole; 2007.

[12] Wechter J, Phillips LJ, Toledo AH, et al. Allopurinol Protection in Patients Undergoing Coronary Artery Bypass Graft Surgery. *Journal of Investigative Surgery.* 2010;23:285-93.

[13] Flikkerma R, Toledo AH, Anaya-Prado R, Toledo-Pereyra LH. Statistical Analysis. *J. Invest. Surg* 2011, 24:237-242.

In: Principles of Research
Editor: Luis H. Toledo-Pereyra

ISBN: 978-1-62417-968-6

Chapter 8

SAMPLE SIZE DETERMINATION

***Robert Flikkema*[1]*, Benedict Dormitorio*[1] *and Luis H. Toledo-Pereyra*[2]**
[1]Western Michigan University, Department of Statistics, Kalamazoo, MI, US
[2]Western Michigan University School of Medicine, Michigan State University College of Human Medicine, Michigan State University College of Osteopathic Medicine, Kalamazoo, MI, US

INITIAL CONCEPTS OF SAMPLE SIZE

One of the most critical yet frequently misunderstood principles of research is sample size determination. Obtaining an inadequate sample is a serious problem that can invalidate an entire study. Without an extensive background in statistics, the seemingly simple question of selecting a sample size can become quite a daunting task. This chapter aims to give a researcher with no background in statistics the basic tools needed for sample size determination. After reading this chapter, the researcher will be aware of all the factors involved in a power analysis and will be able to work more effectively with the statistician when determining sample size. This work also reviews the power of a statistical hypothesis, as well as how to estimate the effect size of a research study, which are the two key components of sample size determination. Several examples will be considered throughout the text.

FURTHER CONCEPTS OF SAMPLE SIZE

The question of sample size is one of the most common yet misunderstood questions in medical and surgical research [1-12]. Oftentimes the researcher approaches the statistician with the idea that the statistician can produce an ideal number of observations to obtain with any given study. In reality, the number of variables involved when determining sample size makes this quite a daunting task. Adding to the complexity of sample size to achieve a desired level of power in a statistical hypothesis test [3, 11]. The researcher and statistician must work together in order to estimate the crucial factors required to determine an appropriate sample size. In this chapter, the main factors involved with sample size determination will be evaluated and incorporated into better defining a new study.

POWER ASSESSMENT

One of the first questions that is typically asked of a statistician is "What sample size do I need?" This seemingly simple and straightforward question is actually incomplete. The driving force behind sample size determination is the power of a statistical hypothesis test. Briefly, power is the chance of a significant statistical test given that there is a significant effect. For example, a certain medical intervention, in reality, increases the survivability of patients. Here, power is the chance that the statistical test will find a significant increase in survivorship of the patients given the sample size used. Thus, researchers generally want to conduct a powerful test in that there is a good chance of detecting a significant effect given that there is an effect.

On the other hand, the amount of statistical power a research has will depend on what type of research is being conducted. A student writing a research paper for a class will need a much smaller power and sample size than a pharmaceutical company testing a new drug. The consequences for an incorrect hypothesis test in the former situation may mean a small markdown in grade, but the latter situation could mean a company investing millions of dollars in an ineffective drug, or throwing out a drug that could help millions of people but was incorrectly deemed ineffective.

TYPES OF ERRORS

Before understanding what power is, you must first recognize the two types of errors possible in statistical hypothesis testing [4]. Let us speak in terms of the pharmaceutical company testing a drug. Drugs can be either effective or ineffective. If an effective drug is deemed effective or an ineffective drug is deemed ineffective, no error is made in testing and the correct conclusion is reached. But if an ineffective drug is deemed effective, then a Type I Error is made in the hypothesis test. Conversely, if an effective drug is deemed ineffective, then a Type II Error is committed. The power of this hypothesis test is the probability of an effective drug being labeled effective. Of course, any researcher desires that the power of the hypothesis test be as high as possible since that reduces the probability of errors in the study and increases the likelihood of identifying significance in a dataset if significance exists. A power of 100% is desirable but usually not attainable in practice since it requires that the entire study population be sampled. In medical research, 80% power has become the standard, although the researcher is free to choose whatever power he wishes. When deciding on an appropriate power, the factors in the next sections should be considered.

EXAMPLE

Suppose that a researcher wishes to compare the reoperation rate of a particular spinal procedure for patients over 40 years old and patients less than or equal to 40 years old. The researcher determines that a chi-square test is appropriate and the desirable effect size (discussed later) is 0.5(1). The researcher now must decide what power level he wants to achieve. How will the selected power level affect the required sample size? The G Power output, including the power curves and necessary sample sizes for various powers, appears in Figure 1.

From this output, we can see that powers of 0.8, 0.95, 0.99, and 0.6 require sample sizes of 88, 145, 205, and 55, respectively. As stated earlier, 0.80 is the standard power level typically used in surgical research; however, the researcher is free to select a high power level if he wishes. If a researcher feels that finding significance is crucial to the quality of the research study, then a higher power level such as 0.95 should be selected. Many other statistical packages such as Minitab, SAS, and R can perform power analysis as well.

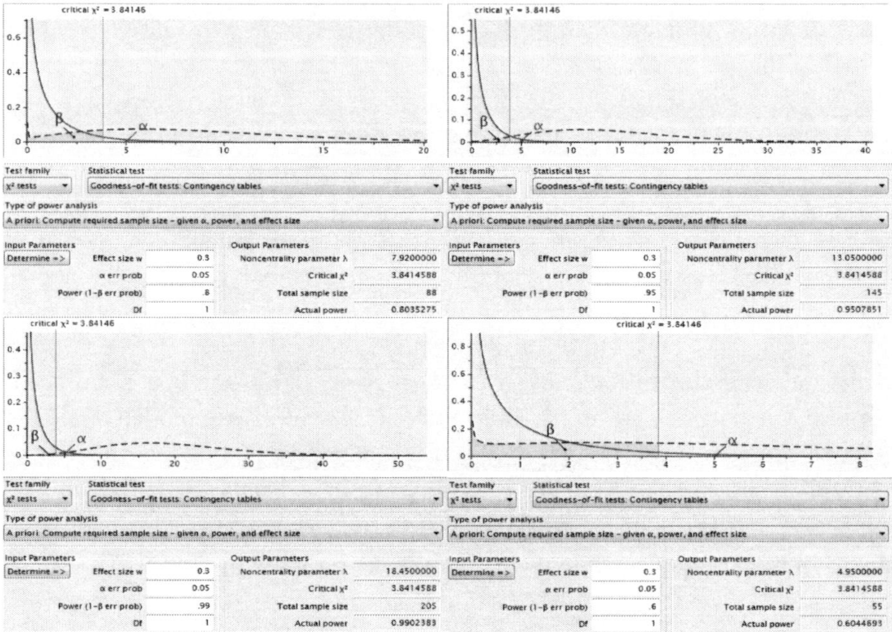

Figure 1. Power curves and necessary sample sizes for various powers.

STRENGTH OF RELATIONSHIP BETWEEN VARIABLES

Another equally important factor in determining sample size is the effect size. Simply, it is the strength of relationship between the groupings of the subjects in the study and outcome [6] and is measured as the ratio of the difference, in means or proportions, of the two groups divided by the standard deviation. A simple example would be if an experimenter is testing for the difference in means between two groups. If the two group means differ only by a small number of standard deviations, the effect size would be small. If the two means differ by a large number of standard deviations, then the effect size is large.

The difficulty in a power analysis is choosing the appropriate effect size. Oftentimes the researcher knows little about the distribution of the data and therefore knows little about the effect size. The researcher must choose an appropriate effect size to test for depending on the desired precision of the study. The intuition between effect size and sample size is that they are inversely related; a large effect size requires fewer samples to detect a significant effect than it would when the effect size is small. If a particular effect size is adequate for a study, then the researcher should not choose an effect size smaller than the one that is adequate since this will cause the necessary sample size to increase substantially. The researcher and statistician need to work together when choosing the necessary effect size of a study.

EXAMPLE

Suppose now that a researcher wishes to determine if there is a difference in the amount of blood loss for a particular type of heart surgery. The researcher plans to use a 2-Sample *t*-test [7] to examine the difference in average blood loss. The researcher decides that she wants 80% power in her study. She now needs to select the effect size that she wants to detect.

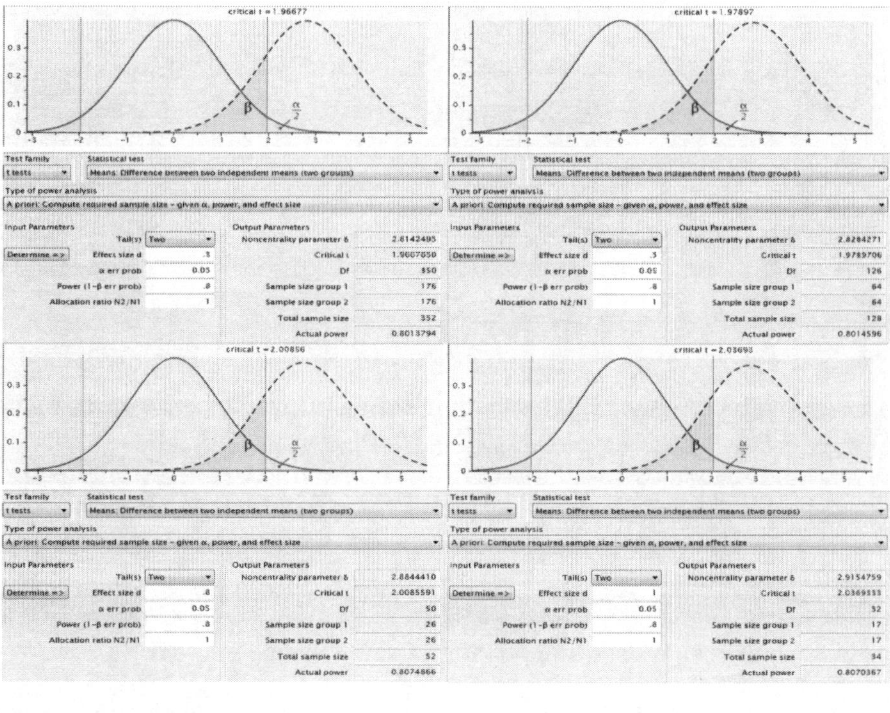

Figure 2. Power and effect size.

We can see from Figure 2 that the effect sizes of 0.3, 0.5, 0.8, and 1 require sample sizes are the sizes necessary for each group, so the researcher would actually have to take double the observations since she has groups of both men and women. From this figure, we can see how choosing the effect size can have a profound impact on the sample size necessary in a study.

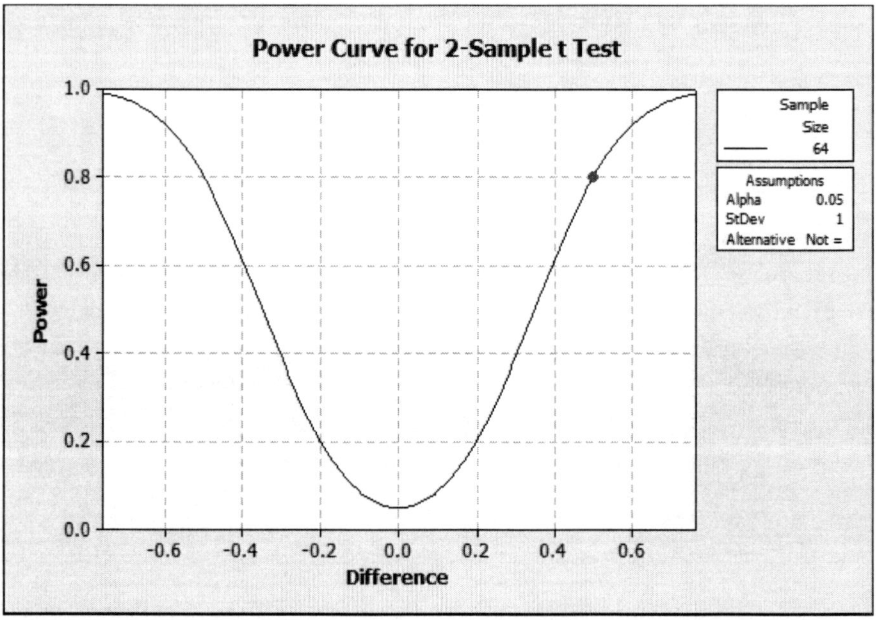

Figure 3. A priori power analysis.

Confidence Level

The confidence level is typically a factor that is not considered, since the 95% level has become so standard in medical research [8]. The confidence level of 95% is equivalent to a significance level of 0.05. This 0.05 is the probability of Type I Error. Going back to our drug example, it means that there is a 5% chance of concluding that an ineffective drug is effective. While the 0.05 significance level is typically sufficient for medical research, the researcher is free to choose the level she wishes. If the results of the study are of special importance, a more appropriate level should be selected.

Sampling Method

In some studies, there are a limited amount of observations available and 80% power simply cannot be achieved. These situations can arise when the cost of taking an observation is very large or there are a small number of people within the study population. With these types of samples, the study can still be run, but the lack of power in the study should be noted and it can prove difficult to find meaningful results.

Power Analysis

Once all of the previous factors are agreed upon, the power analysis can be carried out using statistical software such as R, SAS, Minitab, and G*Power or many other statistical programs. R, SAS, and Minitab are all well-known statistical software packages that perform a variety of statistical analyses. G*Power is a program used specifically to conduct power analysis. An a priori power analysis is run before the data are collected and gives the sample size necessary for the desired power level based on the estimated factors. A post hoc power analysis is conducted after data collection and estimates the actual power achieved by the sample. If one of the previously discussed factors differs from the value estimated by the researcher and statistician, the actual power of the study can differ greatly from the power level selected in the a priori power analysis. If the power was lower than expected, the researcher should explore the option of going back to the population and taking a larger sample. The researcher should always utilize both types of power analyses to ensure that the maximum power level was attained in the study.

Example

Figure 3 is Minitab 16 output for a 2-Sample *t*-test priori power analysis. The power level was at 0.8, while the significance level was set at 0.05. An effect size of 0.5 was used. In this situation, the researcher would need to take a sample size of 64 from each of the two populations in order to achieve 80% power.

CONCLUSION

Sample size determination, although seemed to be a straightforward and an easy problem, involves several factors. For a researcher seeking the help of a statistician, these factors are: 1) effect size, 2) power of the study, 3) confidence level and 4) the sampling method. By presenting these factors in a step-wise and logical manner, this chapter indicates that the researcher and the statistician working together can solve the problem of sample size determination in the most effective way.

REFERENCES

[1] Bartoszynski R, Niewiadomska-Bugaj M. *Probability and Statistical Inference*. 2nd ed. Hoboken, NJ: Wiley-Interscience; 2008.

[2] Chen LM, Ibrahim JG, Chu H. Sample size and power determination in joint modeling of longitudinal and survival data. *Stat Med.* 2011; 30:2295-2309.

[3] Flikkema RM, Toledo AH, Anaya-Prado R, et al. Principles of statistics in surgery. *J Invest Surg*. 2011; 24:237-242.

[4] Hardouin JB, Amir S, Feddag ML, et al. Towards power and sample size calculations for the comparison of two groups of patients with item response theory models. *Stat Med.* Nov 8 Epub, 201.

[5] Mascha EJ, Imrey PB. Factors affecting power of tests for multiple binary outcomes. *Stat Med*. 2010; 29:2890-2904.

[6] Pourhoseingholi MA, Baghestani AR. When calculation of minimum sample size is not justified: When sample size calculation is not justified. *Hepat Mon.*2011;11:208-209.

[7] Rosenkranz GK. The impact of randomization on the analysis of clinical trials. *Stat Med*. 2011;30:3475-3487

[8] Sheskin David J. *Handbook of Parametric and Nonparametric Statistical Procedures.* 2nd ed. Boca Raton, FL: Chapman & Hall/CRC; 2000.

[9] Stallard N. Optimal sample sizes for phase II clinical trials and pilot studies. *Stat Med.* Nov 3 Epub. 2011.

[10] Toledo AH, Flikkema R, Toledo-Pereyra LH. Developing the research hypothesis. *J Invest Surg*. 2011; 24:191-194.

[11] Utts JM, Heckard RF. *Mind on Statistics*. 3rd ed. Belmont, CA: Thomson Brooks/Cole; 2007.

[12] Flikkema R, Toledo-Pereyra LH. Sample Size Determination in Medical and Surgical Research. *J Invest Surg* 2012, 25:3-7.

In: Principles of Research
Editor: Luis H. Toledo-Pereyra

ISBN: 978-1-62417-968-6

Chapter 9

MULTIVARIATE METHODS FOR RESEARCH

***Robert Flikkema*[1], *Benedict Dormitorio*[1], *J. M. Lloris-Carsi*[2] *and Luis H. Toledo-Pereyra*[3]**

[1]Western Michigan University, Department of Statistics, Kalamazoo, MI, US
[2]Universidad Catolica de Valencia, Research Department, Valencia, Spain
[3]Western Michigan University School of Medicine, Michigan State University College of Human Medicine, Michigan State University College of Osteopathic Medicine, Kalamazoo, MI, US

INTRODUCTION

For many medical studies, analyzing a single variable within the population or analyzing multiple variables one at a time is enough to reach meaningful and significant statistical and medical conclusions. However, some studies require an additional level of analysis that goes beyond what simple univariate methods can provide. Multivariate statistical methods allow medical researchers to incorporate multiple variables into a single analysis. This is extremely helpful when there are multiple predictor variables within a population. This chapter will discuss commonly used multivariate methods and how to apply them.

MULTIPLE REGRESSION

A common problem in medical research is when an investigator wants to determine what set of predictors has an effect on an outcome. In this type of problem where the outcome is numeric or continuous, a multiple regression analysis is appropriate. Multiple regression is doubly useful as it not only provides hypotheses tests for each predictor variable as it relates to the response variable, but also provides an equation with slopes or effect for each predictor variable that can be used to determine the expected value of the response variable based on values of the predictor variables. The individual slope of each predictor variable allows the researcher to see if the variable is directly or inversely related to the response variable. Predictor variables with non-significant p-values can be eliminated from the final equation.

When using multivariate regression, it is important to include only uncorrelated predictor variables in the model. Including correlated predictor variables can lead to unreliable results. Correlated predictor variables indicate how well the predictor variables affect the response variables as a whole, but will do a poor job assessing the relationship of each predictor variable individually.

Multiple Regression Equation

$$Y = \beta_0 + \beta_1 z_1 + \ldots + \beta_r z_r + \varepsilon$$

In this equation, Y is the variable being predicted and the z's represent the predictor variables. The betas are calculated using statistical software and indicate how much of an impact each predictor variable has on the response variable.

Multiple Regression Example

Suppose that a surgeon wishes to investigate the operating time of a particular procedure. Specifically, the researcher wants to know if a patient's age, height, and weight can be used to predict the operating time. So our model includes three predictor variables. Fitting the multivariate regression model using the PASW 18 statistical software produces the following output:

Coefficients

Model		Unstandardized Coefficients		Standardized Coefficients	t	Sig.
		B	Std. Error	Beta		
1	(Constant)	122.666	117.309		1.046	.300
	Age	.745	.483	.189	1.542	.128
	Height	-1.046	1.813	-.074	-.576	.567
	Weight	.726	.292	.318	2.491	.016

The Sig. column contains the p-values. We can see that only the weight predictor has a significant p-value. Therefore, we can drop age and height from our final model since they do not significantly predict operating time. Re-fitting the model with just thc wcight prcdictor producccs thc following output:

Coefficients

Model		Unstandardized Coefficients		Standardized Coefficients	t	Sig.
		B	Std. Error	Beta		
1	(Constant)	96.209	22.801		4.219	.000
	Weight	.635	.279	.278	2.278	.026

The coefficients of our equation are found in the B column. Therefore, our final equation is:

$$ORTime = 96.21 + 0.635 * Weight$$

Notice that the weight coefficient is positive. This means that weight is directly related to operating time. Specifically, for each pound a person weighs, a surgeon should expect to spend an additional 0.635 minutes in the operating room.

Logistic Regression

Logistic regression is similar to a multiple regression in that it is used when there is one response variable and at least two predictor variables. On the other hand, a key difference is that logistic regression is used when the response variable is binary. For example, an outcome that is either the presence or absence of disease is a binary outcome. In these sense, a subject in the study can be categorized into one of the two possible outcomes. For simplicity, the two outcomes are usually labeled as 'success' and 'failure.' The success category of the response variable will simply be whichever of the two categories the researcher labels as success. If the response variable is whether or not a person smokes, the researcher could choose to model the probability of a person not smoking, or the researcher could choose to model the probability a person smokes.

Logistic Regression Equation

$$P = \frac{1}{1 + e^{-(\beta_0 + \beta_1 x_1 + \dots + \beta_r x_r)}}$$

The P in this equation is the probability of an observation being a success. The x's in the equation represent the predictor variables and the betas are the coefficients. The value of each beta will determine the influence that each predictor variable has on the probability of success. This equation can be calculated using most statistical software packages.

Logistic Regression Example

In this example, the researchers are interested in examining the effects of a person living alone and type of social support on hospital re-admittance after a procedure. Both the predictor variables are two-category variables and they are predicting the two-category variable of hospital re-admittance. Inputting the data into the PASW 18 statistical software and fitting the logistic regression model produces the following output:

Parameter Estimates

		Estimate	Std. Error	Wald	df	Sig.	95% Confidence Interval	
							Lower Bound	Upper Bound
Threshold	[Readmit = .00]	.439	.545	.647	1	.421	-.631	1.508
Location	[SocialSup=.00]	1.745	.764	5.211	1	.022	.247	3.243
	[SocialSup=1.00]	0	.	.	0	.	.	.
	[LivesAlone=.00]	-.570	.608	.877	1	.349	-1.762	.623
	[LivesAlone=1.00]	0	.	.	0	.	.	.

The first thing to look at in this output is the Sig. column. This column is filled with p-values that tell us if the predictor variables significantly affect the probability of a patient being re-admitted. In this table, the p-value for social support is significant at 0.022, while the lives alone p-value is not significant at 0.349. Therefore, whether or not a person lives alone does not impact if they are re-admitted and we can drop this variable and re-fit the equation.

Parameter Estimates

		Estimate	Std. Error	Wald	df	Sig.	95% Confidence Interval	
							Lower Bound	Upper Bound
Threshold	[Readmit = .00]	.880	.288	9.314	1	.002	.316	1.446
Location	[SocialSup=.00]	1.979	.726	7.422	1	.006	.555	3.403
	[SocialSup=1.00]	0	.	.	0	.	.	.

Now we can get our final equation from the Estimate column. The equation turns out to be:

$$P = \frac{1}{1+e^{-(0.880+1.979*(SS))}}$$

We can see in the table that the beta of 1.979 corresponds to a person not having social support, if a person does have social support, we would set this coefficient equal to 0. Therefore, the probability of a person without social support being re-admitted is 0.946. The probability of a person with social support being re-admitted is 0.707. So our conclusion is that a person having social support significantly reduces their probability of re-admittance.

CANONICAL CORRELATION ANALYSIS

Canonical correlation is used when a researcher wishes to look at multivariate correlation. Specifically, it is used when the researcher has two groups of variables and wishes to determine which pairs of variables between groups have the highest correlation with each other. Since we are dealing with correlation, the variables involved in this analysis must be continuous. Intuitively, this is similar to bivariate correlation analysis using the Pearson correlation coefficient.

Canonical Correlation Example

In this example, the researcher is examining patients undergoing a particular surgical procedure. Three physical and two surgical variables are recorded. The physical variables are height, weight and resting pulse rate. The surgical variables are operating time and recovery time. The researcher wishes to investigate which of the surgical variables are related at all to the surgical variables. The analysis will be run in SAS version 9.2 using the CANCORR procedure.

The CANCORR Procedure

Correlations Among the Original Variables

Correlations Among the Physical Measurements

	Weight	Height	Pulse
Weight	1.0000	0.8556	-0.1169
Height	0.8556	1.0000	-0.0625
Pulse	-0.1169	-0.0625	1.0000

Correlations Among the Surgery Variables

	ORTime	RecTime
ORTime	1.0000	-0.1677
RecTime	-0.1677	1.0000

Correlations Between the Physical Measurements and the Surgery Variables

	ORTime	RecTime
Weight	0.9152	-0.0713
Height	0.8700	-0.0414
Pulse	-0.0419	0.2579

Here are the initial Pearson correlation coefficients between variables. There appears to be strong correlations between the operating time and the weight variable (0.9152), as well as between the operating time and the height variables (0.8700). The recovery time variable appears to have a weak correlation between the three physical variables.

The CANCORR Procedure

Canonical Correlation Analysis

	Canonical Correlation	Adjusted Canonical Correlation	Approximate Standard Error	Squared Canonical Correlation
1	0.938927	0.931832	0.027166	0.881584
2	0.259090	0.172548	0.214016	0.067128

Eigenvalues of Inv(E)*H
= CanRsq/(1-CanRsq)

	Eigenvalue	Difference	Proportion	Cumulative
1	7.4448	7.3729	0.9904	0.9904
2	0.0720		0.0096	1.0000

Test of H0: The canonical correlations in the current row and all that follow are zero

	Likelihood Ratio	Approximate F Value	Num DF	Den DF	Pr > F
1	0.11046657	10.04	6	30	<.0001
2	0.93287233	0.58	2	16	0.5736

Multivariate Statistics and F Approximations

S=2 M=0 N=6.5

Statistic	Value	F Value	Num DF	Den DF	Pr > F
Wilks' Lambda	0.11046657	10.04	6	30	<.0001
Pillai's Trace	0.94871214	4.81	6	32	0.0013
Hotelling-Lawley Trace	7.51679677	18.28	6	18.326	<.0001
Roy's Greatest Root	7.44483873	39.71	3	16	<.0001

NOTE: F Statistic for Roy's Greatest Root is an upper bound.
NOTE: F Statistic for Wilks' Lambda is exact.

The CANCORR Procedure

Canonical Correlation Analysis

Standardized Canonical Coefficients for the Physical Measurements

	Physical1	Physical2
Weight	0.6917	-0.1810
Height	0.3475	0.2005
Pulse	0.0923	0.9859

Standardized Canonical Coefficients for the Surgery Variables

	Surgery1	Surgery2
ORTime	1.0134	0.0431
RecTime	0.1274	1.0063

Notice that the first canonical correlation is larger than any of the between-set Pearson correlations from the previous table. The p-value associated with this canonical correlation is <0.0001. So we can be very sure that this canonical correlation is not 0.

The first canonical variable for the physical variables is a weighted sum of weight (0.6917) and height (0.3475) with more emphasis on weight. The coefficient for pulse is close to 0. We have already shown that pulse exhibits low correlation between the two surgery variables so we can ignore this variable.

The CANCORR Procedure

Canonical Structure

Correlations Between the Physical Measurements and Their Canonical Variables

	Physical1	Physical2
Weight	0.9782	-0.1247
Height	0.9335	-0.0160
Pulse	-0.0102	0.9946

Correlations Between the Surgery Variables and Their Canonical Variables

	Surgery1	Surgery2
ORTime	0.9921	-0.1256
RecTime	-0.0425	0.9991

The correlation between weight and height and the first canonical variable are both positive and quite strong (0.9782 and 0.9335).

To sum up, height and weight have a strong positive relationship with operating time, while the other variables in the dataset are not strongly related.

MANOVA

There are research studies wherein multiple outcomes are studied at the same time. For example, a toxicology study is looking at the effect of a drug on blood pressure, heart rate and EKG parameters at the same time. Also, the researcher wants to take into account the correlation between the outcome variables at the same time. For this type of problem, a Multivariate Analysis of Variance (MANOVA) technique is appropriate. Here, the effect of the groups on multiple outcome variables is assessed at the same time taking into account the inter-relationships between them (correlation between outcome variables.)

MANOVA Example

Suppose that a spinal surgeon is interested in comparing a person's age and opening disc pressure between their discogram morphology, which is classified into three groups. Running the MANOVA in Minitab 16 produces the following output:

The main thing to look at in this table is the Wilk's p-value. This is a p-value testing to see if differences exist between our two variables between the three groups. Our p-value of <0.001 indicates that there are significant differences in our independent variables, but it does not tell us what those differences are exactly. In order to get a better idea of where the differences exist, we can look at the means of the data.

General Linear Model: Age, OP versus Disc Morphology

MANOVA for Disc Morphology
s = 2   m = -0.5   n = 169.0

Criterion	Test Statistic	F	DF Num	DF Denom	P
Wilks'	0.85345	14.017	4	680	0.000
Lawley-Hotelling	0.17163	14.546	4	678	0.000
Pillai's	0.14661	13.487	4	682	0.000
Roy's	0.17119				

Variable	Disc Morphology	Q3	Maximum
Age	ABN	50.250	74.000
	NE	55.00	56.00
	NL	48.000	74.000
OP	ABN	25.00	100.00
	NE	33.75	60.00
	NL	45.00	100.00

So it appears that within the age variable, the NL and NE group means differ, and for opening pressure, the ABN and NL group means differ. If the researcher wanted to further verify which group means are different, a post hoc analysis, such as a multivariate Scheffe' test, could be run.

CONCLUSION

In this chapter, the reader is introduced to four statistical methods which deal with analyzing a relatively large amount of variables at the same time. In summary, when there are at least two predictors to account for, a multiple regression analysis is appropriate when the outcome is numeric and logistic regression is appropriate when the outcome is binary. When there are multiple outcome variables and predictors, a canonical correlation analysis is used to study the inter-relationships between them and MANOVA is used to study the effect of grouping and predictor variables to the outcome variables.

REFERENCES

[1] Bartoszynski R, Niewiadomska-Bugaj M. *Probability Statistical Inference.* 2nd ed. Wiley-Interscience, 2008.

[2] Bhatia R, Wier M. Safety in Numbers, re-examined: can we make valid or practical inferences from available evidence? *Accident; Analysis and Prevention. Oxford: Pergamon Press.* Jan; 34:235-40. 2011.

[3] Cirillo J, Henneberg M. Sequencing human ribs into anatomical order by quantitative multivariate methods. *Homo* 2012, 63:182-201.

[4] Corberán-Vallet A. Prospective surveillance of multivariate spatial disease data. *Stat Methods Med Res.* 2012, 21:457-477.

[5] Flikkema RM, Toledo AH, Anaya-Prado R, Toledo-Pereyra LH. Principles of statistics in Surgery. *Journal of Investigative Surgery.* 24: 237-42. 2011.

[6] Januszyk M, Gurtner GC. Statistics in Medicine. *Plastic Reconstructive Surgery* 127:437-44, 2011.

[7] Johnson RA, Wichern DW. *Applied Multivariate Statistical Analysis. 6th ed.* Upper Saddle River, New Jersey: Pearson Prentice Hall, 2007.

[8] Sheskin DJ. *Handbook of Parametric and Nonparametric Statistical Procedures. 2nd ed.* Boca Raton, Florida: Chapman & Hall/CRC, 2000.

[9] Toledo AH, Flikkema R, Toledo-Pereyra LH. Developing the Research Hypothesis. *Journal of Investigative Surgery.* 24: 191-4, 2011.

[10] Utts JM, Heckard RF. *Mind on Statistics. 3rd ed.* Belmont, California: Thomson Brooks/Cole, 2007.

[11] Valotto G, Quaranta A, Cattaruzza E, et al. Multivariate analysis of Ion Beam Induced Luminescence spectra of irradiated silver ion-exchanged

silicate glasses. *Spectrochim Acta A Mol Biomol Spectrosc.* 2012; 95:533-539

[12] Wu HW, Sturm R. "What's on the menu? A review of the energy and nutritional content of US chain restaurant menus." *Public Health Nutr. Rand Corporation.* 2012; 16:87-96.

[13] Flikkema R, Lloris Carsi JM, Toledo-Pereyra LH. Multivariate Methods in Research. *J Invest Surg.* 2012; 25:203-208.

SECTION II
QUALITIES PERTAINING TO RESEARCH

In: Principles of Research
Editor: Luis H. Toledo-Pereyra
ISBN: 978-1-62417-968-6

Chapter 10

TEN QUALITIES OF A GOOD RESEARCHER

Luis H. Toledo-Pereyra
Western Michigan University School of Medicine,
Michigan State University College of Human Medicine,
Michigan State University College of Osteopathic Medicine,
Kalamazoo, MI, US

Writing about the best "Ten Qualities of a Good Researcher" represents a great responsibility since it is not simple to assemble in a concise manner all the important qualities of a good researcher. Knowing the difficulties lying ahead, I would like to suggest the following qualities: *interest, motivation, inquisitiveness, commitment, sacrifice, excellence, knowledge, recognition, scholarly approach, and integration.* The characterization and understanding of these ten qualities would be extremely helpful to those who are beginning the exciting field of research, and particularly those who will be involved in teaching research.

To be a good researcher first requires the intention to be involved in research and immediately thereafter to show a dedicated interest to do the best research possible [1-4]. From here we must accumulate the knowledge needed to advance the current ideas already existent in the research world. The intention of this chapter is to introduce ten qualities that I consider essential for a good researcher to succeed.

Quality #1: Interest

It is obvious that without interest, desire or disposition towards research we cannot even start thinking about developing some kind of acceptable research. The kind of research is not as important as attempting to get involved in some aspect of it, from thinking of the idea to the different steps involved in completing the process. Interest in research becomes perhaps one of the most important elements since interest is the engine moving the research enterprise further along. One could say, have interest and you can complete the project!

The ideal circumstance would be that the possible trainee has a question that he/she wants to answer and, therefore, research is the conduit for reaching the sought-out level of understanding or offering a well-analyzed response to the question. My advice would be to get interested in research and you will find a universe of worthwhile considerations that satisfy your desire for having appropriate and rational responses.

Quality #2: Motivation

Even though this quality is very close to the previous one of having interest/desire/disposition towards research, it is somewhat different in that motivation takes us one step further to the initial interest reflected towards the research field. One could say that without interest there is no motivation or it could be presented the other way around that without motivation there is no interest.

The dictionary gives an accurate characterization of motivation as "providing for a reason to act in certain way," the equivalent of "inducement, cause, impetus" [1]. In this way, motivation provides the reasoning behind the initial interest in research. It gives the impetus for advancing the initial desire expressed towards the research process. It gives us the inducement for continuing our path of research interest.

Quality #3: Inquisitiveness

This quality is not difficult to introduce since an inquisitive mind is almost a requirement for a good research experience. Without inquisitiveness it would be in many ways impossible to advance the research arena. My advice to the newly initiated in research is to find the ways in which you can advance your questioning one step beyond your current understanding of facts.

Being inquisitive is being curious or, as many dictionaries would describe it, being "unduly curious" (1). Asking frequent questions and showing eagerness for knowledge completes the sphere of the inquisitive mind or the inquisitive individual. In research, this is a fundamental quality that accompanies the initial interest and motivation expressed for research matters.

Quality #4: Commitment

The development of a good research plan or strategy needs commitment to move forward in the completion of the research project. The perseverant hand of the researcher—from the conception of the idea through the required regulatory items and the collection and analysis of the data—is fundamental in the completion of the research study. Remaining committed to the research project is an essential quality in the development and execution of the study. Without commitment, many of the researchers will not be able to progress with the plans needed for the execution of the study. Commitment is the basis for having research clearly available to those interested in this discipline.

Commitment takes the researcher to the end of the planned experiment but at the same time permits the advance of plans for possible publication in a referred journal and/or presentation at a recognized venue.

Quality #5: Sacrifice

The researcher is not only interested, motivated, inquisitive and committed to do research, but is also ready to sacrifice time and efforts in other areas to apply them to his/her research plans and ideas. Without some personal sacrifice it is not possible to create an atmosphere of progress and advancement for the studies being carried out. And this sacrifice will be indispensable in the research work.

Sacrifice becomes an intricate part of the researcher's strategy since it is necessary when using commitment to complete the research operation. Sacrifice is the quality being turned around to finish the study, to complete the quality of the work, to reach excellence whenever possible. Sacrifice enhances the availability of a good research idea being carried through.

QUALITY #6: EXCELLING

When doing research, the researcher should be ready to excel in developing the research idea, the research hypothesis, the experimental design, and the appropriate collection of data. Taking into consideration these various stages of research is fundamental in the completion of the research protocol. One might be able to advance without excellence but cannot reach higher levels without its presence since excellence offers to the researcher the opportunity to obtain results not easily reached before.

Excelling or excellence also applies to the analysis and interpretation of the data, including the writing of the study and its presentation, which will culminate the long hours of dedication to research. I would recommend to the young investigator to think, proceed and mature concepts of excellence, concepts that permit us to improve our profession in the sense that disease will be dominated and patient care improved.

QUALITY #7: KNOWLEDGE

It does not take too much to understand that knowledge is a quality that the researcher cannot do without, since the whole research project depends on it. Knowledge equals advancement, which at the same time equals innovation and discovery (2). It would not be simple to discover without knowledge as much enthusiastic as one might be. Cultivating knowledge represents the most important sphere of the researcher since knowledge lead us to terrains that have not been opened up before.

In order for the research idea to progress, one needs knowledge to support it and eventually move it forward [3, 4]. Knowledge is behind any substantive progress in research. Acquiring knowledge becomes then the main foundation on which research will stand.

QUALITY #8: RECOGNITION

The recognition quality more generally refers to being aware of the research project and how to carry it out and evaluate it. Recognition is needed when the researcher is attempting to maintain a good evaluation path for acquired data and its subsequent assessment. Recognizing the value of the results of the particular project in progress is one of those qualities that one does not see very often until it becomes obvious. We need to instill on the future researcher the value of recognition and how this quality will make results more evident.

Recognizing the research process, how it is evolving, and whether any important developments might be occurring is critical to the research evaluation. Recognition then will be helpful to the researcher who wants to excel on his/her study.

QUALITY #9: SCHOLARLY APPROACH

Once the research project is fully completed, the next step is to assemble it for presentation at a local, regional or national meeting, and eventually to submit it for publication in a peer-reviewed journal of repute. In order to do this, the researcher needs to carefully review his/her data, analyze the literature, and begin the process of writing the manuscript for publication.

If the goal is to submit it for presentation first, an abstract will have to be elaborated in a manner that includes: introduction, rationale, hypothesis, material and methods, results, discussion and conclusion. All these elements will help to secure its acceptance.

The scholarly approach represents, then, the best manner in which a researcher prepares himself/herself to publish or present the data collected and analyzed.

QUALITY #10: INTEGRATION

The integration of all the previous qualities of a good researcher is needed when developing a good research project. A researcher must utilize the various characteristics already mentioned when proceeding to do the best research project possible. Integration of the research process or study is of great magnitude when advancing successfully along the path of research. In this area, collaboration with other researchers or a group of researchers has to be successfully integrated when obtaining results that will be meaningful in clinical or experimental medicine.

Integration can work by helping the researcher to accumulate information obtained from all research stages or by clarifying all aspects of the research. In this way, the researcher will have the best result possible.

Conclusion

The "*Ten Qualities of a Good Researcher*" introduced herein can be considered individually and mainly with the purpose of aiding the uninitiated in the field of research with the ultimate goal of obtaining the best results possible. The best results refer to the planning of a good study, obtaining the most acceptable data, carefully analyzing the results obtained and putting the information together for presentation or publication. At this point, the ten qualities of a good researcher will culminate in obtaining the best publication possible.

References

[1] *Dictionary.Com*, word "motivation" Goggle accessed 6/2/12.
[2] Toledo-Pereyra LH. *Innovation and Discovery on Surgery, History and the Humanities*. Landes Bioscience, Austin Texas, 2009.
[3] Hakim NS. Principles of Research. *Exp Clin Transpl.* 2007, 2:631-632.
[4] Toledo-Pereyra LH. Importance of Medical and Surgical Research. *J Invest Surg*, 22:325-326, 2009.

In: Principles of Research
Editor: Luis H. Toledo-Pereyra
ISBN: 978-1-62417-968-6

Chapter 11

Passion for Research

Luis H. Toledo-Pereyra
Western Michigan University School of Medicine,
Michigan State University College of Human Medicine,
Michigan State University College of Osteopathic Medicine,
Kalamazoo, MI, US

Where to Begin

By now, you have read the previous chapter dealing with the "Ten Qualities of a Good Researcher". There is no question, I believe, that they have motivated you when preparing to be the best investigator possible. In this case, we are adding a special quality that was not necessarily expressed on the previous chapter. This quality is particularly important because without passion or committed enthusiasm for research, a successful career in medical or surgical research is almost unimaginable [1-3]. As a good dictionary would indicate, passion is intense desire, dedicated fervor, and powerful ardor to conquer a particular activity in life. Passion is also great enthusiasm and uncontrollable zeal to excel. Passion suffuses accomplishment, success, improvement, advancement, and all the other attributes of progress. Passion demands our full giving but returns fruits in plenty. In many ways, the disciplines of medical or surgical research are not different from regular life. The medical or surgical investigator needs to build up, encourage, and maintain all the important characteristics of passion. Without passion, medical or surgical research loses its focus on the highest standards of academics and scholarship.

As researchers, we need to teach students and colleagues the enormous benefits of a passionate life, the noble mission of discovering with oriented purpose. Time in the medical or surgical research laboratory should represent the finest time of each day. Entering a laboratory without passion is like diagnosing without a history and physical, performing surgery without knowledge of anatomy, or writing a novel without a plot. Passion drives experimentation, planning, and the pursuit of truth. And passion perpetuates more passion.

Great Examples to Follow for Some Surgeons

Passion has been the immediate source of discipline and methodical exploration in the lives of great scientific surgeons and physicians [1-3]. Consider the contributions of these renowned surgeon researchers: John Hunter (1728-1793) to experimental surgery, Joseph Lister (1827-1912) to antiseptic surgery, William Halsted (1852-1922) to safety in surgery, Harvey Cushing (1869-1939) to brain surgery, Evarts Graham (1882-1957) to lung cancer and gallbladder diagnosis, and C. Walton Lillehei (1918-1999) to open-heart surgery. What about William Osler (1849-1919) the primer internist who advanced the teaching of residents to the highest level of medicine and propagated the use of bedside patient evaluation to establish a good diagnosis? What about Helen Taussig (1898-1986) who created the field of pediatric cardiology at Johns Hopkins Medical School? And, many more that were creators in medicine and surgical matters. Could they have succeeded without their intense passion?

In pursuing medical or surgical research, one should ask, “Is it possible to teach passion to our medical students, young residents and/or faculty?” At first the answer may not be evident. Yet we can reply in the affirmative by remembering that passion can be learned through daily exposure and the continuous example of medical or surgeon masters. Passion grows in the research laboratory that exudes passion and exemplary work. Passion reaches others when there are tangible benefits from its practice. Passion translates into practice when the institution’s leaders, surgery unit directors, and staff thrive on the daily opportunities to foster passion in their specialty and research.

FINAL WORDS

Passion is among the significant factors advancing medical or surgical research, for passion fuels the great advances associated with the discipline in study. Without passion we discover little worth our consideration. Passion directed appropriately, consummates the marriage between knowledge and intuition, between patience and aggression, between understanding and leadership. Passion ignites the whole operation, elevating the enterprise to new triumphs.

The importance of passion – in all the arts and sciences – has been recognized and used to improve endeavors and motivate individuals to fulfill their highest potential. Pursue discovery, act passionately, and judge prudently – this would be my advice to the uninitiated and initiated when entering the prestigious doors of medical or surgical research.

REFERENCES

[1] Toledo-Pereyra LH. Discovery in surgical investigation: The essence of Charles Brenton Huggins. *J Invest Surg*. 2001; 14:251.

[2] Toledo-Pereyra LH. Innovation and Discovery on Surgery, History and Humanities. *Landes Bioscience*, 2009, Austin, TX.

[3] Toledo-Pereyra LH. *Surgical Revolutions. A historical and Philosophical View*. World Scientific, Singapore, 2011.

In: Principles of Research
Editor: Luis H. Toledo-Pereyra
ISBN: 978-1-62417-968-6

Chapter 12

ETHICS OF RESEARCH

***Luis H. Toledo-Pereyra*[1], *Roberto Anaya-Prado*[2] *and Alexander H. Toledo*[3]**

[1]Western Michigan University School of Medicine,
Michigan State University College of Human Medicine,
Michigan State University College of Osteopathic Medicine,
Kalamazoo, MI, US

[2]Health Research Division, Hospital of Obstetrics and Gynecology,
Mexican Institute off Social Security, Guadalajara, Jalisco, Mexico

[3]University of North Carolina, Division of Abdominal Organ
Transplantation, Chapel Hill, NC, US

Ethics began thousands of years ago and can be considered as ancient as philosophy itself. At the very beginning of civilization, early Sumerians recognized the importance of justice and moral principles [1]. With this in mind, they created the Hammurabi Code based on a strict and serious retribution to the surgical damage incurred. Professionals of medicine recognized early on they had to behave on certain manner, a manner that carried consequences if their work was not performed to the expectations placed on them. Physicians and in this case surgeons required to master their art to take care of patients and to accept success or failure on their actions. The discipline of medicine in general has a long history as well, and the study of both medicine and ethics has greatly influenced the practice of patient care and research in medicine.

Medical or surgical research are close and important allies of medicine and surgery themselves [1-8]. Physicians, surgeons and researchers have all united to define and expand themselves the medical or surgical field based on the most advanced modern concepts. Essential to the understanding and practice of medicine and/or surgery is the study of ethics. Apart from ethics, medicine and/or surgery cannot be conceived and appreciated. But even more significant is the application of ethics in medical and surgical research, since these disciplines highlight the importance of experimentation in animals and human beings.

ESSENCE OF MEDICAL AND/OR SURGICAL ETHICS

Essentially, the ethics of medical or surgical research refers to the application of good and reasonable behavior to the best moral care of people and animals, as well as the development and implementation of good laboratory practices in the detailed execution of clinical and experimental studies. To perform sound and acceptable medical or surgical research, the physician or surgeon researcher must adhere to the ethics of the discipline. Executed with the best science available, good research entails a series of stages – the conception of a research project, the ideal care of experimental and human subjects, and the appropriate interpretation of data. The consummation of these stages of medical or surgical research allow for science and ethics to collaborate intimately, thereby achieving the best results.

The principles of ethics – respect, beneficence, justice and autonomy – are all applied to human research. The informed consent obtained without coercion or undue influence is critical within the basis of ethically considered principles. The use of vulnerable populations such as minors, those with illiteracy, pregnant women, prisoners, and the ones with limited access to health care need to be carefully evaluated with special attention to all ethical fundamentals.

Since modern times, when the extraordinary French physiologist Claude Bernard (1813-1878) began experimenting on animal subjects, the use of medical and surgical research have increased exponentially. Bernard's interest in animal experimentation was kindled by his teacher, Francois Magendie (1785-1855), who demonstrated in animals that the spine's dorsal nerve roots were sensory whereas its ventral roots were motor. A significant discovery then and equally important today. Bernard advanced Magendie's work by investigating how these nerve impulses were transmitted and blocked [2]. In

1865, Bernard wrote his monumental work on "*The Introduction to Experimental Medicine*", declaring here that it was appropriate to use animals for research purposes [3]. Later on, he would use animal experimentation to study the effect of substances for mitigation of pain.

EARLY ETHICAL CONSIDERATIONS OF MEDICAL AND SURGICAL RESEARCH

In the Greco-Roman world, Galen (130-200) experimented a great deal with animals. His studies permitted the development of theories and assumptions that practically paralyzed the acceptance of newer concepts until a successful challenge was put forward by Andreas Vesalius (1514-1567) during the Renaissance [4]. William Harvey (1578-1658) and Robert Hooke (1635-1703) engaged in animal research to authenticate their principles of circulation and respiration with sound experiments [4]. These scientists did not consider or present ethical considerations in their research. In fact, no one up to this point had mentioned or even appreciated the role of ethics in animal research. Bernard would be the first to take preliminary steps toward the integration of ethical ideas in animal research with the assertion that pain was not acceptable in the course of animal experimentation, and that anesthesia should be used to lessen its presence [2].

Mitigation of pain became critical to animal research since the times of Claude Bernard. Few years later, if physicians wanted to do research in animals, they had to consider how to protect them. Anesthetics, sedatives and analgesics eventually were the best means to mitigate pain. Being aware of protecting animals from pain had to be the most important ethical principle under consideration.

ETHICS IN ANIMAL RESEARCH

The year 1876 brought animal experimentation to the forefront when the British passed an act regulating the research of animals [2, 5]. How to eliminate pain or animal suffering was the main issue, but the act also stated that animal studies could only be permitted for well-planned research, not for public demonstrations or teaching [2]. This act was the solid foundation for the future ethics of medical and surgical research, but Americans responded unsuccessfully to the challenge. The proposed American legislation (Gallinger Bill) had ideas similar to the British Act, but further emphasized the development of goals, both clinical and physiological, during the research process. This bill did not reach consensus through the legislative process, and its passage was stalled. Organized medicine (eg. The American Medical Association) and medical research groups vehemently opposed this legislation, only to come up with their own guidelines in the early 1900s. These guidelines stressed the living conditions of animals, particularly those conditions under which the experiments were conducted [2].

Several decades later, following World War II, the United States refocused its attention on biomedical research and animal experimentation. Consequently, national policies began to evolve. The Guide for the Care and Use of Laboratory Animals of 1985 (revised in 1996) and the Public Health Service Act of 1986 became the basis for the current guidelines under which animal research is performed in this country [2, 5]. The highest ethical principles were pursued through these regulations. The Office of Laboratory Animal Welfare at the National Institutes of Health supervises the activity of local Institutional Animal Care and Use Committees (IACUCs), securing in this way the utmost standards of integrity in the practice of animal research.

Guidelines Regulating Human Research

In comparison, what are the guidelines regulating the research in human subjects in this country? Notably, the United States regulations are more advanced than the Nuremberg Code and the Declaration of Helsinki. The use of independent review boards (Institutional Review Board (IRB) or the Research Ethics Committee) has improved the conditions of ethics in research, as well as the opportunities for research subject protection. Careful analysis of the research design with emphasis on individual autonomy, and the equitable selection of candidates with optimal risk/benefit ratio, together comprise the basic tenants for the practice of morally acceptable clinical research. In this regard, the U.S. government has developed several offices dealing with research integrity and protection of human research subjects. The Office of Scientific Integrity, now known as the Office of Research Integrity in the Department of Health and Human Services (DHHS), actively participates in maintaining high-quality standards of scientific research. The Office for Protection of Research Risks, now functioning as the Office of Human Research Protection, also associated with the DHHS, is a complementary office oriented to maximizing the opportunity for the protection of human subjects undergoing research. In addition, the Food and Drug Administration (FDA) office of research supervision completes the three necessary government offices that can supervise clinical research in a given moment. However, depending on the project being carried out generally only one of these offices will be involved.

CONCLUSION

In short, the ethics of medical or surgical research should adhere to the most stringent requirements of animal and human protection. Research is second only to the care of human and experimental subjects. Ideally, research and ethics work hand in hand to the development of the most advanced medical and surgical research guidelines. In essence, a physician or surgeon researcher without ethics is unfit to practice the science of experimentation in the medical or surgical field.

REFERENCES

[1] Garrison AH. *An Introduction to the History of Medicine*. 4th ed. Philadelphia: WB Saunders; 1929.

[2] Brody BA. *The Ethics of Biomedical Research. An International Perspective*. New York: Oxford University Press; 1998.

[3] Bernard C. *Introduction to the Study of Experimental Medicine*. New York: Dover Press; 1957.

[4] Lyons AS, Petrucelly RJ II. *Medicine, An Illustrated History*. New York; Harry N. Abrams; 1978.

[5] Orlands FB. Data on animal experimentation in the United States. *Perspect Biol Med.* 1994; 37:217-231.

[6] Toledo-Pereyra LH. *Vignettes on Surgery, History and Humanities*. Landes Bioscience, Georgetown, Texas, 2005.

[7] Toledo-Pereyra LH. American Research Leadership and Ingenuity in Toledo-Pereyra LH. *Vignettes on Surgery, History and Humanities*. Landes Bioscience, Georgetown, Texas, pp. 150-151, 2005.

[8] Arenas-Marquez H, Anaya-Prado R. Errors in Surgery. Strategies to Improve Surgical Safety. *Cir Cir* 2008; 76:355-361.

SECTION III
SCHOLARLY ACTIVITIES: PUBLICATIONS

In: Principles of Research
Editor: Luis H. Toledo-Pereyra
ISBN: 978-1-62417-968-6

Chapter 13

PURSUING SCHOLARLY ACTIVITIES

Luis H. Toledo-Pereyra
Western Michigan University School of Medicine,
Michigan State University College of Human Medicine,
Michigan State University College of Osteopathic Medicine,
Kalamazoo, MI, US

INTRODUCTION

Several years ago, around 2005, the Accreditation Council for Graduate Medical Education (ACGME) wisely considered that all 27 approved residency programs initially leading to board certification, including general surgery, internal medicine, pediatrics, medicine/pediatrics, orthopedics, family medicine, emergency medicine, psychiatry, and many others, should offer evidence of scholarly works. This recommendation was incorporated into the regular standards of educational works such as conferences, bedside teaching, grand rounds, hospital rounds, operating room teaching, and journal clubs. All this would demonstrate that the resident and the associated faculty were progressing at an appropriate pace within the academic scene.

In this regard, the ACGME developed several types of scholarly activities that would permit them to gauge the academic activity of the resident and faculty involved in the teaching of future practicing American surgeons, physicians, and other members of the medical community. This writing defines scholarly activities and analyzes my participation since July 1, 1999 as director of research initially at Michigan State University/Kalamazoo Center for Medical Studies and since July 1, 2012 as director of clinical research at Western Michigan University School of Medicine. We worked on the systematic evaluation of publications first and then other scholarly works at our institution.

Definition of Scholarly Activities

The Merriam-Webster Dictionary defines scholarly works as those "suitable to learned persons" (www.meriam-webster.com/dictionary). In 1638, the value of scholarly works was for the first time considered. In the 1870s, the term research was introduced in England and the United States followed through in 1906 with the support of Daniel Coit Gilman [1], president of the Johns Hopkins University.

On the excellent monograph of Ernest Boyer, "*Scholarship Reconsidered*", published in 1990 at the auspices of The Carnegie Foundation, scholarly activities were placed at the center of academia, research, publications, and teaching [1]. The ACGME demonstrated sound judgment when they apply many of these concepts to the work of residents and faculties on the pursuit of the highest level of academic medical activities [2-5].

Types of Scholarly Activities

The ACGME introduced three types of scholarly activities: (1) scholarly activities of discovery represented by original articles and grants; (2) scholarly activities of dissemination that included review articles, chapters in books, and editorials; and (3) scholarly activities of application integrated by abstracts and presentations at local, regional, and national academic meetings [2-4]. At the end, it is important to mention that scholarly activities are principally publications, in one way or another, except for grants and meeting presentations.

The type of scholarly activities above mentioned would permit to judge the evolution of the resident and to determine if the faculty and program in general were introducing the resident to the world of academics so important in the progression of the particular specialty under consideration [1-8].

SCHOLARLY ACTIVITIES OF DISCOVERY

Original articles and grants represent this particular scholarly activity [2, 3]. It is not difficult to note that this activity is probably the one that involves in general a higher degree of time and commitment to be able to realize its full completion. However, all is dependent on the attention given to the particular scope of the scholarly activity pursued.

Original articles are represented by clinical or laboratory work that deal with unique ideas and principles that respond to hypothesis-driven analysis and fact-oriented work. In this direction, we can see original laboratory work in animals, cells, tests, or theoretical considerations addressing important questions that can be answered in the laboratory scene.

Original articles are also well-represented by clinical studies that by its unique nature offer the opportunity for the resident or faculty of responding to concerns that can only be studied under clinical conditions. In this case, we have several opportunities for study, especially those based on prospective studies, retrospective studies, and surveys. The depth of each one of them would vary depending on the problem and nature of the question in study and the extension in which the idea is being pursued.

Prospective studies generally represent fresh data and analysis of new findings generated by testing a *de novo* hypothesis, by defining the extension of the results, and by integrating an organized response. Retrospective studies analyze charts of patients with events that occurred in the past, with circumstances that already happened, and with phenomena that we already know from history. This kind of project can offer a great deal of information and depending on the data and analysis of it, one can obtain very much worthwhile information. The surveys are as valid and meaningful as the questions asked and the information received. In this regard, surveys can represent a very positive resource of consideration for the researcher who is serious about defining his/hr data better and advancing the knowledge of that particular item on study. It is then from our point of view that there is no better type of study than others, but rather how the study was planned and conducted so that we can reach the major benefits after its execution.

Grants are generally hypothesis-driven, and the time spent on their elaboration is proportional to the difficulty of the goals sought for within the frame of the study. Federal grants such as the National Institutes of Health (NIH) type are time consuming and require elaborate planning on their completion. Even though with this preparation, less than 15% or so are successful, that is are fully funded. Other types of grants at the local or state level require less time and are more frequently funded. The investigator at this point needs to decide about the direction to pursue based on the possibilities of success and funding for his/her work. Another type of grant not frequently rewarded with funding is the one associated with medical, surgical, or various other societies that offer the opportunity to obtain funding with less onerous commitment on time and resources. The faculty or resident will need to decide about the type of grant in which he/she can invest all the needed time to be successful.

Scholarly Activities of Dissemination

Review articles and chapters in books represent this particular scholarly activity [2, 3]. Both require time commitment and opportunity to finish the task. The time commitment is proportional to the depth on which the project is reviewed and analyzed.

Review articles are as complicated or simple as the other articles in the different categories. They must include, by definition, a great deal of information and be authored by individuals who have experience on the particular area of interest. Both requirements are needed, extensive literature review and author's knowledge and previously publication on the field. The review article can give a great opportunity to the author to expose his/her points of view and claim new ways of thinking, new theories or hypotheses depending on the specific areas studied. The review article, in another way, is a good manner for the recently initiated resident or faculty to expand their knowledge at the same time that they have the opportunity to publish. The only unsolicited requirement is to have as the senior author a well-known expert on the topic to be reviewed.

Chapters in books are necessary when teaching residents and faculties the extensive details of the specialty. However, there is no simple way to have the opportunity to write them but to be associated with faculty that already is participating on writing chapters within their regular activities of the residency. This important scholarly activity can only be accomplished if the faculty is committed to searching for new pathways on the world of book publishing.

Scholarly Activities of Application

Abstracts and presentations at recognized local, regional, national, or international meetings constitute this particular scholarly activity [2,3]. The degree of scholarly commitment is clear when reviewing these functions. First, some kind of acceptable work needs to be completed prior to abstract submission. Second, acceptance is required prior to presentation. The two then integrate a good combination to excel in scholarly activities of application.

Abstracts must be organized in a specific manner to be considered for publication. To learn how to write the successful abstract is essential. Faculty needs to participate with residents on the completion of the good abstract. It is clearly important that residents learn how to write the best abstracts for submission. Attention to detail is worth considering it when assembling the data for abstract writing.

Presentations at academic meetings are critical to the development of the resident or faculty. Both require to excel in presenting their works to advance their specialty knowledge. Specific aims should be directed ad being clear, logical, with good visual aids, following time constraints, and having a well-prepared conclusion. A good presentation can improve the understanding of the topic and represent an asset for the residency program and the institution behind. Good presenters are physicians or surgeons that can clearly communicate and have patients who can understand their point of view. Good communication is a great asset for daily clinical activities.

Integration of All Scholarly Activities

All scholarly activities are important, none being superior to the other. On the contrary, all of them complement each other. On the contrary, all of them complement each other. To have a part of each one of the three scholarly activities is perhaps the best form of accomplishment. To concentrate in one but not in the others probably is not as ideal, but it is not, in anyway, penalized by the regulating body, the ACGME.

There are no numbers required by the ACGME as the best quantity recommended. There is no combination required as well. There is no mentioning that a combination of the three scholarly activities is needed either. What is important most likely is to have some form of scholarly activities present. Residency programs would be better evaluated if the scholarly activities can demonstrate how the residents and faculties maintain a scholarly environment. Below we can indicate the language most frequently used by the ACGME.

Scholarly Activities According to ACGME[1]

The ACGME recommends the following:

1. "The curriculum must advance resident's knowledge of the basic principles of research, including how research is conducted, evaluated, explained to patients, and applied to patient care."
2. "Residents should participate in scholarly activities."
3. "The sponsoring institution and program should allocate adequate education resources to facilitate resident involvement in scholarly activities."

ACGME Scholarly Activity Requirements [2].

Scholarly Activities at Michigan State University/Kalamazoo Center for Medical Studies until June 30, 2012 (and on July 1, 2012 the Institution was Renamed to be Western Michigan University School of Medicine [WMed])

For several years, since July 1, 1999, when I arrived at Michigan State University/Kalamazoo Center for Medical Studies (now WMed), we have maintained a registry of all faculty publications. Figures 1-3 demonstrate the evolution of publications in peer-reviewed journals, chapters in books, and book editorships[2] at our institution since my arrival. Figure 4 introduces the

[1] All activities can be further specified by the Residency Review Committee.

[2] Represents all the elements included in publications only such as peer-reviewed publications, chapters in books, and book editorships. The rest are represented in scholarly activities as mentioned before and have been defined above.

number of scholarly activities including the number of publications as presented above in addition to grants, abstracts, and presentations. All the authors were represented by faculty, full-time, part-time, and occasionally a community faculty. Residents by themselves without faculty were rarely considered in this group. The number of faculty in the institution has varied slightly through the years with approximately 60-65 (1999-2010) annual faculty members

It is evident that our faculty has remained very competitive regarding the number of publications during this period of time. The reasons why we have so significantly increased the number of publications is not debated in this work, but suffice it to say that the combination of continuous encouragement from the Research Department, appropriate allocation of education resources including the support of a statistician, and if needed a grant, and/or manuscript writer, and other research endeavors associated with an academic financial incentive program were all determinants of the success we have seen so far (Figures 1-4).

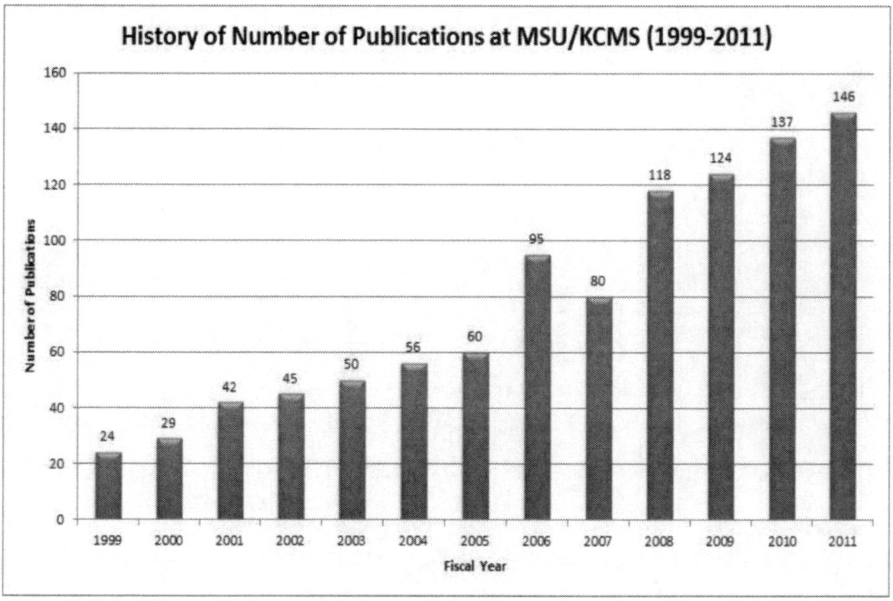

Figure 1.

By the time the ACGME decided to formally institute the theme of scholarly activities in 2005 as the basis for recognizing the academic output of residents and faculty [2], we were readily prepared to deal with this new development. In this way, our change was prompt and fully incorporated into our academic numbers (Figure 4).

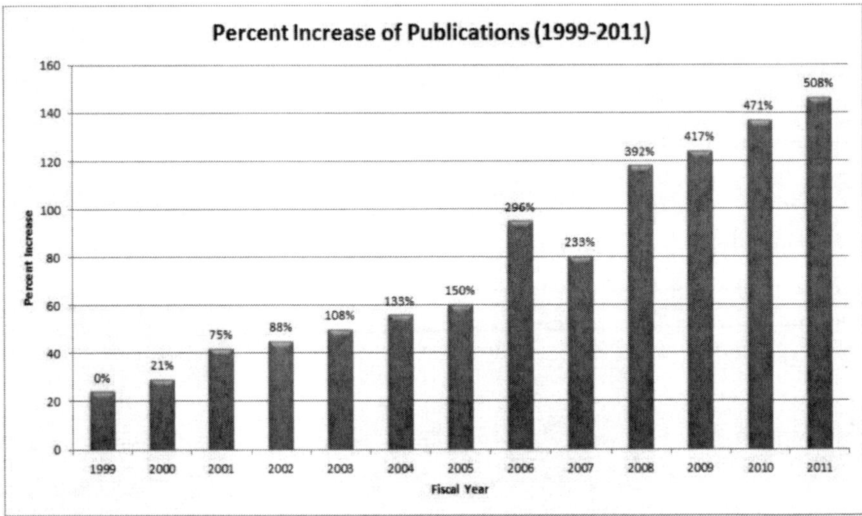

Figure 2.

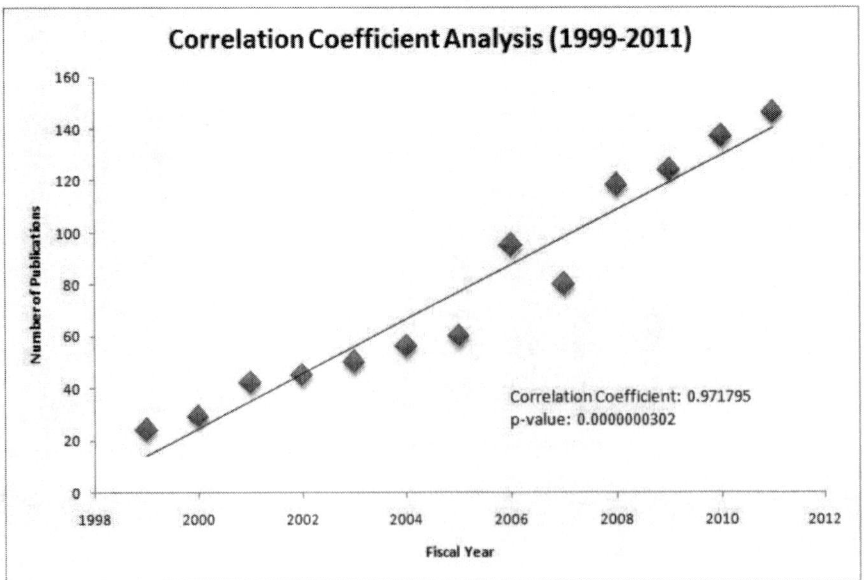

Figure 3.

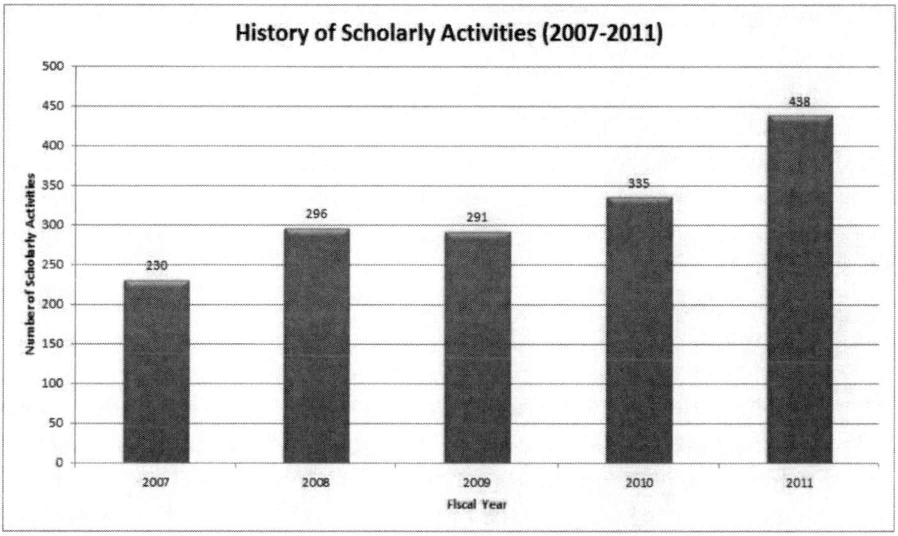

Figure 4.

Figures 1 and 2 shows the number an percentage increase of publications, respectively. For the percentage increase, the comparison is to 1999, which is the first time registered by us. Figure 3 introduces the correlation coefficient analysis for all these publications[2] as presented in Figure 1. Figure 4 presents the evolution of the scholarly activities sine its reporting at our institution in 2006-2010 as incorporated by the ACGME. In brief, the difference between Figure 1, which only represents peer-reviewed publications, chapters in books, and book editorships[2] and Figure 4 is the addition of grants, abstracts, and presentations to Figure 1. Summarizing, scholarly activities are then represented by publications as given by peer-reviewed publications, chapters in books, and book editorships plus the new addition of grants, abstracts, and presentations. In either one, the old system of publications only or the new system with scholarly activities [2-4], the numbers continue to progressively increase as more faculty participation is incorporated into the subsequent reports.

PERSONAL OBSERVATIONS

As I had the opportunity to report on the academic output of our faculty starting on July 1, 1999, and continuing through my 13th year today in 2012, I have observed some interesting developments that are the key to improved results and are worth to consider them here:

1. I believe that communication with and support of the faculty and residents are the most important ingredients of success. Taking the principle that research is a service department and that faculty and residents are our customers, we must be available at all times to attend their needs in our academic setting.
2. Now, after overcoming our previous hurdle, we needed to build a relationship with our faculty, including those who are strong publishers as well as those who do not publish that much and are starting to learn the ways of improved scholarly works. Any opportunity to create a positive atmosphere cannot be wasted, and it should always be utilized.
3. Gaining the trust of the faculty is vital for a Research Department and for increasing publications since all decisions will reflect in any possible manner how the faculty was better supported.
4. Including the faculty on any decision made that might affect them in one way or another was very important when building a strong pattern of support.
5. Utilizing the Research Committee as a way to communicate with the faculty and gain their respect and appreciation for your work remained a great value undertaken.
6. Developing other subcommittees or research groups that might help on the overall positive response of the faculty and staff was important. Communication again was incorporated in the evolution of these working groups. The most crucial of these small groups was the one integrated by faculty who wanted to discuss philosophical, historical, and humanities problems. It was called the "Clinical Research Scholars" Group.
7. Advancing the participation of faculty, especially on the activities of the Research Day, which is the annual scholarly gathering of faculty, residents, and medical students where all, after acceptance, presented their works.
8. Respecting and protecting faculty, as much as possible, on the development and elaboration of the scholarly activities.
9. Giving presentations to residents and faculty on how, where, and what research is all about was of great help.

10. Finding ways to help faculty, residents, and medical students was essential to reaching their attention when matters of scholarly works were discussed and taken into consideration by most of those involved in academics.

After everything had been said and done, scholarly activities were more swiftly moved ahead with the support of the Chief Executive Officer of the institution. Having the participation and support of Dr. Robert P. Carter initially (from my beginning in 1999 until June 2008) and Dr. Elizabeth A. Burns later on (from July 2008 to 2013. In July 2012, the institution became WMed and Dr. Burns continued as Associate Dean of Faculty and Clinical Affairs) was extremely important since residency program directors were more in tune with his/her communication in the efficient overall development of the scholarly works.

The incorporation of a financial incentive program for faculty involved in scholarly activities, practically since my arrival in 1999, was very helpful and served to stimulate various members of our staff. I do not believe that this incentive program on its own was the dominant element on the improvement of scholarly activities but was extremely encouraging.

Conclusion

Many factors participate on the continuous increase of scholarly activities in an institution with 10 allopathic and 3 osteopathic residency programs and a total of 201 residents today, namely communication, trust, support, respect, and financial incentives of the publishing faculty. Teaching and support of residents as to how to do and implement research are also of considerable importance. Supporting medical students can be worthwhile when incorporating them into the entire research enterprise.

References

[1] Boyer EL. *Scholarship Reconsidered*. New York: The Carnegie Foundation for the Advancement of Teaching; 1990.

[2] *Graduate Medical Education Directory* 2005-2006, 90th ed. Chicago, IL: AMA Press; 2005.

[3] *Graduate Medical Education Directory* 2008-2009, 93th ed. Chicago, IL: AMA Press, 2008.

[4] *Graduate Medical Education Directory* 2010-2011, 95th ed. Chicago, IL: AMA Press, 2010.

[5] Glassick CE, Huber MT, Maeroff GI. *Scholarship Assessed.* New York: The Carnegie Foundation for the Advancement of Teaching; 1997.

[6] Toledo-Pereyra LH. In the Pursuit of Scholarly Activities. J Invest Surg. 2010, 23:335-341.

[7] Toledo-Pereyra LH. *Reminiscences on Surgery, History and Humanities.* Landes Bioscience, 2007, Austin, TX.

[8] Anaya-Prado R, Toledo AH, Toledo-Pereyra LH. The Surgeon as Scientific Writer. *J Invest Surg* 2006, 19:335-339.

In: Principles of Research
Editor: Luis H. Toledo-Pereyra
ISBN: 978-1-62417-968-6

Chapter 14

FOSTERING SCHOLARLY ACTIVITIES AND PUBLICATIONS

Luis H. Toledo-Pereyra
Western Michigan University School of Medicine,
Michigan State University College of Human Medicine,
Michigan State University College of Osteopathic Medicine,
Kalamazoo, MI, US

INTRODUCTION

Scholarly activities and publications go hand-in-hand with the positive progression of academic life. The development of a systematic approach to scholarly activities will permit a better outlook for publications, presentations, and grants. In this way, scholarly activities represent the essential part of the academic arena. Without scholarly activity, there is no advancement in academics. Thus, fostering scholarly activities and encouraging publications would be crucial when developing the academic faculty of the future.

Scholarly activities nourish academic productivity and vice versa. Equally important, academic development is based on scholarly activities. The most important denominator of scholarly activities is publications. Without them, the academic world would not progress as expected. In this work, we review the best means to fostering scholarly activiti8es and encouraging publications [1-10].

What Are the Most Important Elements of Scholarly Activities?

When fostering scholarly activities, the first element is the research environment and the interest and commitment of administration and faculty. The environment conducive to research represents a significant advancement when reaching the most scholarly oriented goals.

A good environment, with the inclusion of the elements that are required to complete the research project, is necessary. The availability of an infrastructure for clinical pharmaceutical trials and the assistance of research coordinators would be helpful. The support and effective partici8pation of a well-structured Research Committee, an Institutional Review Board (IRB) and/or Privacy Board (PB) necessary to complete the research.

As mentioned before, the dedication of the faculty – even though sometimes difficult to realize because of their clinical commitment – is a very important part of the process. The administrative support is important as well, especially when providing the positive support and encouraging the faculty to advance on the research ladder. A helpful hand from the research team facilitates the overall path to research completion and eventually to publication.

How Do We Collect Information and Maintain Confidentiality?

During the process of research protocol approval, the Collection Data Sheet is fully discussed and approved by the appropriate committees. In this regard, details of what is important for the hypothesis and aims of the experiment are considered, discussed, and approved. The collection of information is then carried out as promptly as needed for the study. Maintaining confidentiality during the collection of information, storage, and use of data becomes an issue of extreme concern since the significance of patient protection and confidentiality cannot be over-emphasized and must be respected at all times. Once the information has been gathered and responses have been reviewed as previously addressed by the aims of the study, and the literature has been reconsidered, the actual writing of the study results begins. Special attention should be directed to the right venue for publication. Careful analysis of the best journal for publication, suited for the results obtained, must be considered when preparing the paper for publication. The information obtained will then be written in accordance to the directions for authors.

THE ACTUAL PUBLICATION

Once the data have been collected and the journal (or any other site for publication) h has been selected, the preparation of the paper should follow the guidelines provided by the journal. These should be clear, concise, and right to the point. In scientific work, statistics will be a significant part of results and conclusions. In general, the publication should include the title page (authors and affiliations); the abstract (1 page or less); the introduction (2/3 of a page); materials and methods (where the statistical analysis should be described; the results, and finally, the discussion (3-4 page), where the review of the literature will be introduced in relationship to the results observed in the study. At the end, the conclusions should be presented in 2 to 3 sentences at the most. After this, the references should be included. The figures and tables will be added after the references, but have been previously referred to within the paper.

CONCLUSION

Scholarly activities and publications are basic elements of academic accomplishment. Therefore, fostering scholarly activities and encouraging publications are at the center of a complete academic life.

REFERENCES

[1] Toledo-Pereyra LH. In the pursuit of scholarly activities. *J Invest Surg* 2010; 6:335-341.

[2] Wood BP, May W. Academic recognition of educational scholarship. *Acad Radio.* 2006; 13:254-257.

[3] Raff BS, Arnold J. Faculty development: an approach to scholarship. *Nurse Educ.* 2011; 26:159-161.

[4] Levine RB, Hebert RS, Wright SM. Resident research and scholarly activity in internal medicine training programs. *J Gen Intern Med.* 2005; 20:155-159.

[5] Fincher RM, Work JA. The scholarship of teaching in health sciences schools. *J Vet Med Edu.* 2005; 32:1-4.

[6] Sabir M, Penney DG, Remine SG, Mittal VK. Scholarly activities-essential to surgical education. *Curr Surg*. 2003; 60:459-462.

[7] Mavis B, Katz M. Evaluation of a program supporting scholarly productivity for new investigators. *Acad Med.* 2003; 78:757-765.

[8] Willis DR, Kelton M, Saywell RM Jr, et al. An incentive compensation system that rewards individual and corporate productivity. *Fam Med* 2004; 36:270-278.

[9] Andreae MC, Blad K, Cabana MD. Physician compensation programs in academic medical centers. *Health Care Manage Rev*. 2006; 31:251-258.

[10] Brandt TL, Romme CR, LaRusso NF, et al. A novel incentive system for faculty in an academic medical center. *Am Inter Med.* 2002; 137: 738-743.

SECTION IV
REGULATORY FUNCTIONS OF RESEARCH

In: Principles of Research
Editor: Luis H. Toledo-Pereyra
ISBN: 978-1-62417-968-6

Chapter 15

CLINICAL RESEARCH COMMITTEE APPROVAL

Luis H. Toledo-Pereyra
Western Michigan University School of Medicine,
Michigan State University College of Human Medicine,
Michigan State University College of Osteopathic Medicine,
Kalamazoo, MI, US

Clinical Research Committee approval (CRCA) is required at our institution. In other institutions, the approval of the Institutional Review Board (IRB) is sufficient. The rationale for recommending Clinical Research Committee approval prior to IRB approval relies on the fact that since we are an intricate part of a medical school, we take pride ourselves of educating our medical students and residents in how to write a good research study. In addition, we utilize the time of preparing the Clinical Research Committee application as an opportunity to develop the formal IRB submission. And, finally, we maintain a well-organized record of all studies being carried out and approved at our medical institution and therefore knowing who obtains CRCA facilitates a great deal our mandate.

There is another aspect that needs to be introduced into the logic of requesting a separate Clinical Research Committee approval before IRB consideration, and that is the absence of separate scientific review approval by some IRBs for principal investigator initiated research. In this regard, even though the federal regulations indicate: "The federal regulations under which

IRBs operate, however, do not clearly call for IRB review of the scientific validity of the research design" (*Institutional Review Board Guidebook*, Chapter IV, Consideration for Research Design, 1993; obtained from hhs.gov/ohrp/archive/irg/irg_chapter4. Accessed on 4/7/2011), however, we seek to take the safest road and request CRCA. It is within this spirit that we emphasize the need for satisfactory review of the scientific analysis of the research study [1,2].

It is worth clarifying that the Clinical Research Committee approval is not a substitute for the IRB approval. The Clinical Research Committee approval is an institution requirement and can change, be modified or eliminated at any time depending on institution goals and development; whereas, the *IRB is under federal regulations and therefore essential within approval process.*

REFERENCES

[1] Lind SE. Innovative Medical Therapies: Between Practice and Research. *Clinical Research* 36:546-51, 1988.

[2] *Institutional Review Board Guidebook.* Office of Human Research Protection, Health and Human Services, 1993.

In: Principles of Research
Editor: Luis H. Toledo-Pereyra
ISBN: 978-1-62417-968-6

Chapter 16

INSTITUTIONAL REVIEW BOARD (IRB)

Luis H. Toledo-Pereyra
Western Michigan University School of Medicine,
Michigan State University College of Human Medicine,
Michigan State University College of Osteopathic Medicine,
Kalamazoo, MI, US

The Institutional Review Board was developed to "assure that the rights and welfare of patients or research subjects were protected" [1]

Important considerations related to the development, function and activity of IRBs are: [1]

- They originated from two abuses of human subjects: 1. Nazi physicians experiments of World War II, and 2. Tuskegee Syphilis Study on black American men from Alabama between 1932 and 1972 sponsored by the U.S. Public Health Service.
- The IRBs are under United States government mandate, regulated by the Food and Drug Administration (FDA) and the Department of Health and Human Services (DHHS) Office for Human Research Protection (OHRP).
- The IRBs are governed by Title 45 Code of Federal Regulations (CFR) Part 46. Also, Title 21, Part 56.
- The "Common Rule" applicable to IRBs refers to "The Federal Policy for the Protection of Human Subjects" and was adopted in 1991 (45

CFR 46A.) It sets requirements for IRB membership, function and criteria for approval. It defines the general requirements for informed consent, among other functions such as, additional protection for vulnerable research subjects (pregnant women, *in vitro* fertilization, fetuses, prisoners and children).

- The National Research Act was signed on July 12, 1974 referring to the definition and characterization of IRBs, and creating the National Commission for the Protection of Human Subjects of Biomedical and Behavioral Research, active until 1978.
- The IRBs follow the Belmont Report which identified the ethical principles introduced by the National Commission after a four-day conference in February, 1976 in Belmont, Maryland. These principles included: respect for persons, beneficence and justice and were published by the National Commission in 1979.
- The IRB composition must includes at least five members with experience on the ethical considerations of research, familiar with vulnerable populations, at least one non-scientist, one scientist and one community member. It is also important that members exclude themselves from voting on their projects. This IRB group reviews and approves the observances of good ethical principles associated with clinical studies. The scientific basis of the clinical study is often reviewed by the Scientific Studies Committee that in our institution we call it, Clinical Research Committee, and we have referred to it in a previous chapter. Other IRBs review on their own the scientific approval of the proposal even though is not a general mandate of the "Common Rule".
- Since the approval of informed consent is essential to the function of the IRBs, it would also be important to add in this section the "Elements of Informed Consent" that so clearly and comprehensively have been described on the FDA (Food and Drug Administration) Code of Federal Regulations.

FDA Code of Federal Regulations
FDA Good Clinical Practice
2011 Reference Guide
As of April 1, 2011
Obtained from Clinical Research Resources, LLC
Philadelphia, 2011
(Documents in the public domain, not copyrighted)

§50.25 Elements of Informed Consent

a *Basic elements of informed consent.* In seeking informed consent, the following information shall be provided to each subject:

1. A statement that the study involves research, an explanation of the purposes of the research and the expected duration of the subject's participation, a description of the procedures to be followed, and identification of any procedures which are experimental.
2. A description of any reasonably foreseeable risks or discomforts to the subject.
3. A description of any benefits to the subject or to others which may reasonably be expected from the research.
4. A disclosure of appropriate alternative procedures or courses of treatment, if any, that might be advantageous to the subject.
5. A statement describing the extent, if any, to which confidentiality of records identifying the subject will be maintained and that notes the possibility that the Food and Drug Administration may inspect the records.
6. For research involving more than minimal risk, an explanation as to whether any compensation and an explanation as to whether any medical treatments are available if injury occurs and, if so, what they consist of, or where further information may be obtained.
7. An explanation of whom to contact for answers to pertinent questions about the research and research subjects' rights, and whom to contact in the event of a research-related injury to the subjects.
8. A statement that participation is voluntary, that refusal to participate will involve no penalty or loss of benefits to which the subject is otherwise entitled, and that the subject may discontinue participation at any time without penalty or loss of benefits to which the subject is otherwise entitled.

b *Additional elements of informed consent.* When appropriate, one or more of the following elements of information shall also be provided to each subject:

9. A statement that the particular treatment or procedure may involve risks to the subject (or to the embryo or fetus, if the

subject is or may become pregnant) which are currently unforeseeable.

10. Anticipated circumstances under which the subject's participation may be terminated by the investigator without regard to the subject's consent.
11. Any additional costs to the subject that may result from participation in the research.
12. The consequences of a subject's decision to withdraw from the research and procedures for orderly termination of participation by the subject.
13. A statement that significant new findings developed during the course of the research which may relate to the subject's willingness to continue participation will be provided to the subject.
14. The approximate number of subjects involved in the study.

b When seeking informed consent for applicable clinical trials, as defined in 42 U.S.C. 282(j)(1)(A), the following statement shall be provided to each clinical trial subject in informed consent documents and processes. This will notify the clinical trial subject that clinical trial information has been or will be submitted for inclusion in the clinical trial registry databank under paragraph (j) of section 402 of the Public Health Service Act. The statement is: "A description of this clinical trial will be available on http://www/ClinicalTrials.gov, as required by U.S. Law. This Web site will not include information that can identify you. At most, the Web site will include a summary of the results. You can search this Web site at any time."

c The informed consent requirements in these regulations are not intended to preempt any applicable Federal, State, or local laws which require additional information to be disclosed for informed consent to be legally effective.

d Nothing in these regulations is intended to limit the authority of a physician to provide emergency medical care to the extent the physician is permitted to do so under applicable Federal, State, or local law.

[45 FR 3690, May 30, 1980, as amended at 76 FR 270, Jan. 4, 2011]

§50.27 Documentation Of Informed Consent

a Except as provided in §56.109(c), informed consent shall be documented by the use of a written consent form approved by the IRB and signed and dated by the subject or the subject's legally authorized representative at the time of consent. A copy shall be given to the person signing the form.

b Except as provided in §56.109(c), the consent form may be either of the following:

1. A written consent document that embodies the elements of informed consent required by the §50.25. This form may be read to the subject or the subject's legally authorized representative, but, in any event, the investigator shall give either the subject or the representative adequate opportunity to read it before it is signed.
2. *A short form* written consent document stating that the elements of informed consent required by §50.25 have been presented orally to the subject or the subject's legally authorized representative. When this method is used, there shall be a witness to the oral presentation. Also, the IRB shall approve a written summary of what is to be said to the subject or the representative. Only the short form itself is to be signed by the subject or the representative. However, the witness shall sign both the short form and a copy of the summary, and the person actually obtaining the consent shall sign a copy of the summary. A copy of the summary shall be given to the subject or the representative in addition to a copy of the short form.

   [46 FR 8951, Jan. 27, 1981, as amended at 61 FR 57280, Nov. 5, 1996]

References

[1] *Institutional Review Board Guidebook*. Office of Human Research Protection, Health and Human Services, 1993.

In: Principles of Research
Editor: Luis H. Toledo-Pereyra

ISBN: 978-1-62417-968-6

Chapter 17

INSTITUTIONAL ANIMAL CARE AND USE COMMITTEE (IACUC)

***Sylvia Gografe*[1] *and Elysse Orchard*[2]**
Comparative Medicine, Veterinarian Services, Florida Atlantic University, Boca Raton, FL, US
Animal Resources, Small Animal Imaging Center, Louisiana State University Health Sciences Center, Shreveport, LA, US

HISTORY OF THE INSTITUTIONAL ANIMAL CARE AND USE COMMITTEE (IACUC)

In 1961 the Animal Care Panel (ACP) was formed by a group of veterinary research scientists who published the first edition of the Guide for the Care and Use of Laboratory animals in 1963. The most recent revision, the 8th edition (*the Guide*) was published in 2011 and adopted in 2012 as the guiding document for animal care and use supported by the Public Health Service (PHS) and the Association for Assessment and Accreditation of Animal Care International (AAALACi). (See References at the end of the chapter.)

In 1966 the news media published reports on animal neglect mobilizing the public to support the passage of what is now known as the Animal Welfare Act providing minimum legal standards for the care and use of laboratory animals.

In 1971 the policies developed by the National Institute of Health (NIH) and PHS sought to assure that NIH supported research or teaching using live animals met minimum standards of care. The options for carrying out the assurance process allowed for accreditation by an independent accrediting organization of research professionals (now known as AAALACi) or the establishment of an institutional animal care committee to assure animal welfare standards utilizing *the Guide*. The committee composition was not delineated, but it did require that one member be a Doctor of Veterinary Medicine.

In 1979 the PHS Policy was revised to require each grantee institution to maintain "a committee to maintain oversight of its animal care program" and to submit an Assurance statement that PHS supported animal research and facilities would be committed to follow *the Guide*, the Government Principles and the PHS policy requirements. The Assurance further required the committee to be comprised of 5 members, one a veterinarian and whose members were knowledgeable of the care and use of animals used in research.

In1986 the revised PHS Policy required that the members of the Institutional animal care and use committee to be appointed by the chief executive officer of the institution. The AWA amended in1985 required that a member representing the community interests and not affiliated with the institution be appointed to the IACUC.

Humane animal care and use is the purpose and function of the IACUC. The development of the laws and regulations that created the IACUC influenced the composition and contributed to the improved care and oversight of laboratory animals is a dynamic process that will evolve with increasing scientific knowledge, globalization, cultural awareness and training.

AUTHORITY, COMPOSITION AND FUNCTIONS OF AN IACUC

Each institution registered as a research entity with USDA/APHIS and/or receiving Public Health Service (PHS) support for activities involving mammalian or vertebrate animals, respectively must operate an animal care and use program with clear lines of authority and responsibility. This program must include procedures for self-monitoring, an adequate veterinary care program, an occupational health and safety program, a personnel training program, a species specific housing and management program for animals, and most importantly an IACUC. The IACUC is the regulatory unit for animals used in research, teaching and testing in an organization. The constitution of an IACUC is mandated by the Health Research Extension Act and Animal Welfare Act. The Chief Executive Officer of an institution, i.e. the highest official of an organization has to appoint the IACUC members. The CEO, however, may delegate this authority to the Institutional Official (IO). The IO must be a senior administrator who has by virtue of the position the ability to commit institutional resources to ensure compliance with laws and regulations, but is not required to have animal research experience. Each option, whether the IO is an experienced research animal user or not, has its own set of challenges that will be addressed throughout this chapter. The IACUC reports to the IO and more importantly has an advisory role to the IO. This includes guidance on the Institution's compliance with the governing laws and regulations as well as committing the resources needed to correct deficiencies identified. The IACUC is expected to make recommendations to the IO regarding all aspects of the animal care and use program.

The Animal Welfare Regulations (§2.31(a) AWR) and PHS Policy concurrently state that the IACUC must be qualified through the experience and expertise of its members to assess the research institution's animal program, facilities, and procedures. The AWR mandates that at least three members and the PHS Policy that no less than five members compose the IACUC. Both regulations agree on a Chairperson, a Doctor of Veterinary Medicine and an IACUC member non-affiliated with the research facility. The PHS policy requests in addition one practicing scientist and a nonscientist to be appointed to have a fully constitutional IACUC.

It is understood that the Chair is a knowledgeable and effective leader. The person must have sufficient stature in the institution, i.e. has seniority or tenure, to best perform the function of the IACUC Chair and of course needs the full support of the IO.

The Veterinarian is required to have training or experience in laboratory animal science and medicine. Both PHS Policy and AWR mandate a veterinarian to serve on the IACUC with direct or delegated program responsibility. Delegated responsibility in this regard means if a veterinarian is hired on a consulting basis rather than as a full time employee often applicable to very small animal research programs.

The non-affiliated member is commonly referred to as the community member and cannot be connected with the institution in any way other than as an IACUC member. Even further, this person cannot be a member of the immediate family of a person affiliated with the institution. This member is intended to represent general community interests. Due to the introduction of a non-institutional perspective to the research endeavor, this member when well informed brings a significant value to the committee.

The nonscientist's expertise lies in a nonscientific area and again brings a very unique perspective to the committee for not being familiar with animal research models. Often people such as lawyers, members of the clergy, ethicists, accountants or librarians can be found serving in this IACUC member category.

The scientist member is almost self-explanatory and should be experienced in research involving animals. When a research proposal or topic is under consideration the scientist member can provide a valuable perspective. If the scientist member(s) or other IACUC members are not familiar with a specific research topic or concern the IACUC can take advantage of a consultant with the expertise needed. The consultant can provide guidance but cannot function as an IACUC member, i.e. vote.

Alternate members may be appointed to the IACUC. There has to be a one-to-one designation of members and alternates in regards to the role (i.e. scientist, non-affiliated member etc.) but not in regards to a person per se. It is important to note that IACUC members and their respective alternates may not count toward a quorum at the same time.

One member may serve in more than one category as long as the committee has the minimum required number of members. However, this may leave the IACUC at a higher risk of not being properly constituted if an unexpected vacancy in membership occurs. Not all members have to be present at an IACUC meeting as long as it is constituted as per regulatory requirements and a quorum is achieved for tasks requiring a vote. A quorum is defined as the majority, i.e. more than 50% of the members present.

The IACUC is one of the most active committees of a research institution due to its multitude of tasks even in organizations with a smaller animal research program. Moreover, the IACUC is usually the entity that obliges the institution's compliance in areas that appear not to be obvious IACUC terrain, e.g. occupational health and safety, controlled substances use and confirmation of congruency between grant proposals and IACUC protocols. Although done in conjunction with other administrative units it is often a logical result that the animal care and use committee follows through on the aforementioned matters. Federally mandated functions are established similarly in the PHS Policy and the AWR.

The IACUC has to review the institutions animal care and use program for the humane care and use of animals. This review must be performed at least once every six months and includes all components of the program such as IACUC membership and functions, IACUC records and reporting requirements, investigating and reporting animal welfare concerns, veterinary care, IO responsibilities and communication with stakeholders of the program, training of IACUC members, animal care personnel and research personnel, disaster planning and preparedness, occupational health and safety of personnel as well as personnel security.

Once every six months the institution's animal facilities must be inspected. This involves a site visit of the traditional animal housing facilities but also areas where experimental, especially surgical procedures are performed when located outside the vivarium. The site visit team will inspect the soundness and functionality of physical plant components and primary animal enclosures, environmental parameters in the animal housing facilities, regular as well as weekend and holiday care of animals, environmental enrichment, behavioral and social management of animals, cleanliness and sanitation, pest control, waste disposal, recordkeeping, appropriateness of feed and bedding amongst others. Special considerations specific for areas where surgeries, imaging, behavioral studies and other specialized experiments are performed will be assessed.

The evaluation of the facilities and the program review is based on applicable regulations such as AWR and PHS policy. The Guide for the Care and Use of Laboratory Animals is often used since this provides useful details. However, other federal and state regulations need to be considered when applicable. Although inspections of field study sites are not required IACUCs need to be aware of circumstances under which studies are conducted to be able to evaluate the impact on the study subjects, i.e. wild animals and the risks for personnel that may arise. The IACUC has to ensure that appropriate permits have been secured by the study personnel.

The IACUC must prepare and submit reports to the IO to apprise the IO of the state of the animal care and use program and communicate deficiencies found. The report must distinguish between major and minor deficiencies with a specific plan and timeline attached to each deficiency showing the anticipated resolution. It is advisable to meet in person with the IO especially if major resources are needed to correct insufficiencies. The IACUC is responsible for making recommendations to the IO regarding all aspects of the animal care and use program in the organization including but not limited to facilities and personnel training. It is crucial that the IACUC is able to communicate the importance of particular aspects of the program and where improvements are needed especially if the IO is not a researcher trained in the use of animal models.

One of the most important duties of the IACUC is to review and investigate concerns regarding the animal care and use program. There must be an easily accessible mechanism for concerns to be brought forward anonymously or in person to key stakeholders (IO, AV, IACUC administration) of the program without the fear of retaliation. The concerns may result from reports on noncompliance received from animal care personnel, researchers or their staff, employees of the institution or from public complaints. It is imperative to investigate those concerns thoroughly to assure the welfare of the research animals as well as to keep the public trust and support of the ethical and humane care and use of these animals.

Any experimentation conducted using animals covered by the AWR or supported by the PHS must be described and justified by the Principle Investigator (PI). Most institutions decide to have all vertebrate animal research activities described in an animal care and use protocol, commonly known as the IACUC protocol. The IACUC will review the protocol and can approve it, require modification in, or withhold approval. No one, not even the IO can override the IACUC's decision in this regards. The AWR requires review of animal associated activities no less than annually and each IACUC protocol must undergo a denovo review after 3 years.

The same review procedure is applied for significant changes proposed to an approved IACUC protocol. No work can commence until full approval has been granted to an amendment to a protocol. The outcome of the IACUC's review of an amendment can be approval, require modification in, or withhold approval. The PHS provides guidance on what they consider significant changes and it is advised that the IACUC define in a policy/SOP what could constitute a significant change.

In addition to the IACUCs responsibility to investigate and review concerns regarding the animal care and use program it is also responsible for monitoring research projects after approval. If a noncompliance, is detected the IACUC is authorized to suspend an activity involving animals if other measures contemplated would not suffice. This austere action has to be preceded by review of the matter at a convened meeting of the IACUC. A quorum needs to be present to vote on the suspension. The IACUC has to communicate the reasons for the suspension to the IO who must review it, take appropriate corrective action in consultation with the committee and report the detailed incidence to the applicable agency such as OLAW, USDA/APHIS and granting agency. The IACUC can lift the suspension when the committee is certain that remedial actions have led to the resolution of the concern and recurrence of the problem is not likely.

The IACUC like any other regulatory unit or entity of public stature has to be above any conflict of interest either real or perceived. It is stated in both the AWR and the PHS Policy that no member "may participate in the IACUC review or approval of an activity in which that member has a conflicting interest except to provide information requested by the IACUC". That is not limited to being personally involved in a research activity described in an IACUC protocol. It could apply to a member's involvement in a potentially competing research study or that a member is knowledgeable about funding or intellectual information providing an unfair competitive advantage. It would be advisable to abstain from voting when a strong personal bias would interfere with the member's impartial judgment. Parts of this are true for the IO as well. Although not a voting member of the IACUC the IO has the authority to make major decisions that will impact the animal care and use program. It requires an integer personality to surmount the often perceived conflict of interest when an IO is an active animal user while the IACUC and the Attending Veterinarian as a key player of the program report to her/him.

CHALLENGES FACED BY A CONTEMPORARY IACUC

As with any other committee, the IACUC's strength and effectiveness depends on the personalities, integrity and stamina of its members and certainly how well it is supported by the higher administration. The IACUC eventually reflects the overall culture of the institution based on priorities set forth for the research conducted and the relative importance of particular components of the animal care and use program. Sometimes IACUCs are primarily focused on protocol review not only because it is undoubtedly a major component of the committee's work and time consuming but also necessary to avoid delaying studies involving animals. However, establishing and implementing policies tailored to the needs of the particular organization and therefore influencing the culture of an institution to open opportunities for eventually improving animal welfare is as significant as well.

Decisions made by IACUC members are based upon very complex interactions between science, economics, global and organization specific cultures and deeply ingrained traditions that drive the societal ethic. One example is how one looks at different species used as animal models. Does it mean if a society is not valuing certain rodent species as much as companion animals such as dogs and cats that those less regarded species deserve less respect? Or, that swine a species that provides food for humans would feel less anxiety or pain than do nonhuman primate species? Of course, the committee members know that this is not true but nevertheless will be influenced by this perspective of the society. Another matter playing along the same venue is the subject of phylogeny. Species at the upper end of the phylogenetic ladder such as nonhuman primates are thought to be more sentient and possess higher cognitive functions. Human nature is to anthropomorphize and IACUC members are no exemption. The phylogenetic position of the species is a common factor being considered in the review process of study proposals as was reported involving sixty subjects acting as members of a hypothetical IACUC. More and more research is being performed on animal consciousness, self-awareness, cognition and emotions across phylogenetic levels and IACUC members will definitely have to consider this new knowledge in their decision making process independent on which animal species will be used in research and teaching.

A recent survey found that the IACUC is highly regarded as the gate keeper assuring animal welfare. One key concern of the committee is to review study proposals including experiments that cause or have the potential to cause pain and distress and if unavoidable its minimization. This plays into the concept of the "3R's", refinement, replacement and reduction, which need to be considered during the protocol review process. Members of the IACUC now pay attention to the justification why animals cannot be replaced by *in vitro* methods and how animal numbers have been calculated based on statistics. Big strides have been made during the last couple of years in regards to refinement, replacing invasive procedures such as exploratory surgeries by non-invasive procedures such as *in vivo* imaging, the latter being less stressful and particularly less painful for the animal.

Training of all personnel using or caring for animals cannot only promote the understanding of the concept of the "3R's" but is an integral part of the refinement. Training is even often referred as the last frontier in animal research. Here really enormous leaps can be achieved. It makes a huge difference on the post-operative recovery of an animal if the surgeon is experienced and well trained. Skills such as atraumatic tissue handling and strict aseptic technique will have a tremendous influence on the outcome of the surgery minimizing or avoiding pain and infections, respectively. Aseptic technique is not only important for surgical procedures but also post-surgical care of chronic implants. Many research technicians are not medically trained and therefore sometimes lack the understanding of the basic principles of these procedures. Therefore, research personnel needs to be taught about the why and how good surgical and aseptic technique improves the well-being of animals used in surgical models.

Another imperative training topic is species-specific behavior. This is necessary to be even able to assess the pain and/or distress level of an animal during experimentation and eventually provide supportive care appropriate to the species. One needs to know if an animal is naturally timid or gregarious, sedentary or active, social or solitary. How animals express themselves will be influenced by the fact either they are prey species or predators. Prey species often hide pain to avoid being an easy target in the wild. This kind of reaction will not change in confinement. Research personnel needs to be knowledgeable about physiological specifics of the species and how is it influenced by the housing, care and experimentation. An example of this is when an experimental paradigm prevents acoprophagic animal from expressing this behavior, which could lead to nutritional deficiencies over time. Furthermore, it is imperative to be able to address the aforementioned questions to find meaningful and effective humane end-points for a particular animal species and research study. This will allow removing an animal from a study or euthanizing it at an earlier time point to fulfill the mandate for humane and ethical research using animal models.

Training by and collaboration with an expert such as a veterinarian or experienced biological scientist will afford researchers the opportunity to choose the right animal model. Mice have become the species of choice because of the ability to manipulate their genetic material. Genetically engineered mice express or lack biological factors under investigation, carry human genes, can be "humanized" and develop diseases that are actually human ailments and naturally would not inflict their own species. In addition, mice are small, relatively easy to maintain in captivity, very prolific and a mammalian species. Although the small size poses its own challenges especially in surgical models it definitely provides great advantages in resource expenditures including space and husbandry provision as well as in the amount of experimental materials and compounds needed. However, resource conservation should not be the determining factor for selecting the model. Mouse models even when genetically manipulated have limitations and cannot answer all scientific questions. There are species specific physiological characteristics that differ from human physiology and may not be appropriate for the study goals. Of course, this is not only true for mice but for all species and needs to be carefully considered by the IACUC members when reviewing research proposals. To be able to translate results from biomedical research into human applications one has to use the right species. But what is the right species? There is no quick or perfect answer to this, rather one has to study the species in question in depth, consult experts, scrutinize the literature and sometimes learn by trial and error. For the latter a pilot study may be the most appropriate way to achieve the scientific goal while minimizing the number of animals until one can convince the members of the IACUC that a good animal model has been found.

"The IACUC is obliged to weigh the objectives of the study against potential animal welfare concerns." This quote from the 8th edition of the Guide sums up the expectations that the IACUC assess each animal care and use protocol regarding procedures that may cause pain and distress by performing an analysis of the implied benefit (the significance of the proposal) vs. the potential for pain and distress that would be experienced by the animal during the course of the experimental procedures. The PHS and Government Principles are not too different.

When protocol review involves surgical procedures and the investigator states that the use of analgesia will interfere with the aims of the study, the IACUC is faced with an ethical dilemma. Public support for animal research declines proportionally as the pain level increases. Multiple references in the literature on the effect of analgesics on physiology and behavior have been published. The effect of analgesic use must be considered against the physiological effects of pain, which may include impairment of bowel motility and immune suppression. There is sufficient evidence to show that lack of pain control can cause greater impact on the normal physiology and immune suppression than would be expected if analgesia had been provided. Studies have also shown that when acute pain is not controlled there is an increase in chance for chronic pain which would continue to have an impact on the outcome and goals of the study. For the same reasons that the use of anesthesia is considered a requirement for the conduct of survival surgery, the administration of analgesia should be given the same ethical cost/benefit consideration. This is especially true for anesthetic agents that do not have analgesic properties upon regaining consciousness. Isoflurane and pentobarbital two commonly utilized anesthetics are two which are not considered to have any residual analgesia upon recovery.

One of the justifications often stated for withholding analgesics is that the most commonly used effective pain medications will interfere with the study objective since they also possess anti-inflammatory properties. So do a variety of other compounds and drugs, which are sometimes proposed to be used in the same study. The evaluation of agents administered to animals requires very specific expertise, which neither the researcher nor the IACUC members might have. In a case like this it would be advisable to exercise the right to seek advice from a consultant. A pharmacologist for example will be able to weigh in on the effect of a drug and its duration on a physiological process of interest.

If analgesia cannot be provided based on a solid scientific justification the IACUC needs to consider a range of other measures provided by the research staff that can comfort animals when experiencing pain or distress. Supportive care including but not limited to offering a warm, quiet and clean environment, palatable food as well as ease of access to feed and water can help to alleviate pain and anxiety. Companionship by other animals or humans is another example of improving the comfort level. In addition, it behooves the members of the IACUC to request appropriate intervals for monitoring and have humane end-points described in the protocol that are meaningful for the animal, particular experimental procedure and study outcome.

There are many more difficult situations and decisions the committee members have to face during discussions and fulfillment of all their essential functions. This text is only meant to be a snapshot but makes clear that IACUC's should not accept what was acceptable many years ago. Human beings are creatures of habit and one gets used to things being confronted on a regular basis. IACUC members are no exemption. It might be advisable to have a checklist that reminds the committee members during their deliberations to consider things such as phylogeny, cultural perspectives, the right animal model, analgesia, supportive care, frequency of monitoring, appropriate training of personnel and cost-benefit-ratio. The latter meaning the balance between the cost of the animals suffering and being euthanized at the end of the study and the benefit of gaining knowledge relevant to society.

In a number of institutions the IACUC has mastered a huge cultural shift with the result of improved animal well-being and subsequently better science. It will be a continuing effort to challenge the status quo since change is not always welcome. Consequently, a properly functioning IACUC with the overall goal of fostering animal welfare, supporting excellent research and protecting the institution depends on excellent relationships between all stakeholders. Ensuring humane and ethical care and use of animals is based on a partnership between the IACUC, the investigators and their research staff, the veterinarian(s) and animal care staff and certainly the IO and each party carrying their share.

REFERENCES

[1] *Institutional Animal Care and Use Committee Guidebook,* available at http://grants.nih.gov/grants/olaw/GuideBook.pdf

[2] *The Guide for the Care and Use of Laboratory animals 8th ed,* available at http://grants.nih.gov/grants/olaw/Guide-for-the-Care-and-Use-of-Laboratory-Animals.pdf

[3] *Methods and Welfare considerations in Behavioral Research with Animals* http://www.nimh.nih.gov/research-funding/grants/animals.pdf

[4] *Recognition and Alleviation of Pain in Laboratory Animals* http://dels-old.nas.edu/animal_pain/report.shtml

[5] *The Guide for the Care and Use of Agricultural Animals in Research and Teaching* http://www.fass.org/docs/agguide3rd/Ag_Guide_3rd ed.pdf

[6] *Guidelines for the Care and Use of Mammals in Neuroscience and Behavioral Research* http://grants.nih.gov/grants/olaw/National_Academies_Guidelines_for_Use_and_Care.pdf

[7] *OLAW Guidance,* available at http://grants.nih.gov/grants/olaw/faqs.htm

[8] Silverman J, Baker SP, Lidz CW. A self-assessment survey of the Institutional Animal Care and Use Committee, Part 1: animal welfare and protocol compliance. *Lab Animal* 41:230-235, 2012.

[9] Newcomer C. Behold! The animal care and use Magician! AAALAC Connection 10-11, available at http://www.aaalac.org/publications/Connection/ Where_is_the_institution.pdf

[10] Silverman J, Suckow MA, Murthy S. *The IACUC Handbook* 2nd ed, CRC Press, Boca Raton, FL. 2007

[11] *Information Resource for IACUC members and staff,* available at http://www.iacuc.org/index.htm

In: Principles of Research
Editor: Luis H. Toledo-Pereyra
ISBN: 978-1-62417-968-6

Appendix I

BRIEF "GUIDE TO RESEARCH"

Luis H. Toledo-Pereyra
Western Michigan University School of Medicine,
Michigan State University College of Human Medicine,
Michigan State University College of Osteopathic Medicine,
Kalamazoo, MI, US

Dr. Carter Brooks, from our institution, authored *Introduction to Research* (*Getting Started in Research*) which was used in great part as the basis for this Appendix. Dr. Alan Davis and his colleagues from the Grand Rapids Education and Research Center allowed us to utilize their writings from "Present and Publish" at the end of this Appendix.

INTRODUCTION

Research provides an organized approach to answering questions and enhancing knowledge. As such it is a means to an end, not an end in itself. If answers exist for all of your questions you have no need of research. However, as your clinical data bank grows fuller you may find questions for which you haven't any answers because nobody has the answers. Research aimed at addressing these questions can contribute to your clinical competence as well as enhancing the total body of medical knowledge. Even if you have no intent of pursuing a career as an investigator, involvement in the research process will help you evaluate and appreciate the results of others' efforts.

Traditionally those with an ultimate goal of credibility as a researcher will begin their career as an apprentice to a more experienced mentor with an ongoing line of investigation. This pattern can work well at Western Michigan University School of Medicine (WMed), though we are happy to support a trainee's independent line of research if it is well thought out and can be accomplished with the facilities and resources available here. We encourage you to develop a field of special interest which may lead to fellowship training and subspecialization, or at least to intellectual satisfaction. As you become more familiar with a narrower field, gaps in existing knowledge will appear and suggest productive areas for research.

Over the span of one medical lifetime, conducting clinical research has become a much more complex process. Only a few decades back one could take an idea almost directly to the bedside. The investigator was presumed to view the study subject ethically and responsibly, and the potential study subjects seemed to have a higher level of trust in a physician investigator than exists today. This allowed research to proceed rapidly and directly, and most of the time the assumptions of fair and ethical treatment were justified.

But not always. Classical cases of abuse of the process included the Tuskegee study of the natural history of syphilis which denied its participants penicillin treatment that had become available after the study commenced. This made some sense scientifically but was a poor deal for the patient denied a treatment or information about a treatment already generally accepted as effective. Occurrences of this sort plus an evolving sense of rights, responsibility, privacy and more has led to a level of complexity in the research process which many might argue is excessive but has a mandate on multiple levels and determines how we operate.

The steps in the current process are not always intuitively obvious. Often we find students or residents with a good research idea who fail to budget enough time to move the potential project from concept to practice. This guide will outline activities, mostly obligatory, which one must accomplish before enrolling human subjects in a new research study. Of particular use to the prospective researcher, we provide an estimate of the time that should be budgeted to accomplish each step. A few of these activities can occur in parallel but most are sequential with all that implies for time allotment. The number of people and/or departments which review and approve (or not) even a simple research proposal is large and seems to continue to grow.

The bottom lines for a successful project are:

- Avoid unnecessary complexity in design. Ask and answer one question (though several variables may impinge and need consideration.)
- Budget ample time to allow completion of all required activities.

Before You Begin

Research Process

Research Process

From the moment the topic is defined with its multiple variables, the researcher creates an atmosphere that permits to formulate the research question and to develop the hypothesis and specific aims. The research design comes next with the characterization of the statistical analysis. After approval, the data is collected and evaluated prior to final assessment and submission for presentation.

Research Mentor

- Assist in formulating a research question
- Assist in identifying important variables to consider
- Advise patient recruitment/selection process and data collection
- Faculty sponsor for Institutional Review Board (IRB) application
- Co-author presentations/publications

Resident/Fellow in Research

The resident/fellow in research will search the literature, write the protocol, meet several times with the research mentor, and define the goals of the study. From there, the resident/fellow, aided by the mentor, will submit the protocol to the Clinical Research committee and IRB, and begin the project.

Role of Program/Research Director

- Create environment conducive to and supportive of research
- Monitor and facilitate progress of learners' research

- Facilitate communication with mentors and Clinical Research Department
- Assist in review of presentations and manuscripts

Role of Clinical Research Department

Function as a service center for consultation and assistance with:

- Idea/protocol development
- Research design
- Resource identification
- IRB compliance
- Statistical analysis
- Recruit and develop faculty mentors

Timeline for Research

Table 1. Estimates for Protocol Time Requirements

Activity	Time Required
Background information collection	Variable but allow ample time. No less than 1 month
Create hypothesis and study design for testing	Variable – allow 2 weeks
Statistical consultation	1-2 weeks
Revision based on peer review	Variable – at least 2 weeks
Draft final protocol and write Informed Consent	2 weeks
Internal Western Michigan University School of Medicine Clinical Research Department review	2 weeks
IRB Review	4 weeks

Other Activities

- Obtain necessary research certifications (Western Michigan University School of Medicine Clinical Research Office, NIH Human Protection, CITI, Financial Conflict of Interest)
- Obtain funding, if needed

- Identify/arrange for study site
- Plan for study personnel, if needed

The previous table includes activities required to prepare for a study with estimates of the time necessary to accomplish each. These estimates presume no serious time-consuming complications. In some cases more than one activity may be addressed simultaneously which can condense the time requirement a little. These numbers do not include "inactive time" when the project is superseded by other more pressing problems. It appears that under the most favorable of circumstances several months will elapse between the birth of an idea and the IRB approval of a study plan based on that idea. Only at this point can you begin any real study-related activities such as recruiting potential research subjects, followed by evaluation and imposition of study-related variables.

REQUIRED TRAINING

1. ALL learners including faculty, residents and students must complete the NIH tutorial, *"Protecting Human Research Participants."*
   Go to: http://phrp.nihtraining.com/users/login.php
   After you have completed the tutorial you will receive a certificate of completion. Print and submit your certificate to the Western Michigan University School of Medicine Clinical Research Department.
   Record your username and password here for future reference:
   Username: ____________________________________
   Password: ____________________________________
2. ALL researchers must also complete the Net Learning module *"Privacy Rule (HIPAA) for Researchers."*
   From the Western Michigan University School of Medicine intranet, log in to Net Learning, choose 'Enroll in CBL' from the menu on the left side of the page and select the course. Once you have passed the module, your completion certificate will be forwarded from HR to the Research Department.
3. Another important document to be completed is the CITI research approval or the NIH Human Protection internet site approval.

How to Get Started

Research Idea Development

Identify and ask the Critical Question - One of the most important tasks for you and your mentor is the formulation of a clinically important research question.

A question can be generated from:

- An observation made while rounding
- A review of the medical literature
- Grand rounds discussions
- Interactions with peers, colleagues and attendings

Let's suppose that you are interested in allergen sensitization, the allergens involved and the sources of these allergens. You know the allergens which might be encountered under various circumstances out of doors and those which will impact a patient indoors and around various furnishings in these settings. One possible source of allergens on which you can find little information is allergen exposure in an automobile, aside from what might blow in through an open window. Since many of us spend a good part of our life in a motor vehicle this may have some importance as regards development and expression of allergic disease.

This categorical question leads to a long list of related inquiries which might influence how one chooses to design the research project. A partial listing of possibly related (but probably confounding) questions follows:

- What to sample? Interior air, upholstery, carpet, child seat?
- What method(s) to use for sampling and assay?
- Age of the car? Mileage on the car?
- Model of car—minivan, SUV, sedan, convertible, truck?
- Make of car?
- What kind of upholstery or interior finish has the car?
- Is the car air-conditioned?
- Who typically rides in the car?
- Is the car neat or littered inside? Littered with what?
- Do pets ride in the car?
- Where is the car stored when not in use?

- What besides people may be carried in the car?
- Are you looking for any particular allergen?
- Is the car driven predominantly in city, suburbs, rural area?
- Geographic area in which the car is used—Northeast, Southeast, Midwest, etc?
- Has the car always been used in this same area?
- How often is the car washed and/or cleaned inside?

One might ask other questions as well, but *what we need is not more but fewer inquiries*. Remember the desirability of simplicity.

Let's rein in our curiosity and concentrate on occurrence of house dust mites in car upholstery (fabric only) in cars at least two years old. Limit sampling to sites east of the Mississippi River comparing one set from the northern tier of states and another from the southern tier.

Literature Search

Examine Prior Relevant Experience - No matter what research question you choose, you must perform a thorough literature search for your study to:

- Determine the novelty of your research question
- Develop the background or significance section of your proposal
- Gain a better understanding of your topic
- Avoid duplication research
- Avoid errors made in similar research
- Determine how your research can add to the existing body of knowledge
- Obtain ideas to help refine/amend your research question
- Compare/contrast your findings
- Acquire new ideas for methods, definitions, and/or outcome variables that you can use for your study

Never waste your time or resources doing research that someone else has already done, unless you suspect error in the results or conclusions of the prior work. In such circumstances you may set out to verify the earlier report, possibly employing an improved methodological approach. To assure that your intended project represents a novel effort, you must thoroughly research prior art and science in the intended field of inquiry. A few minutes with *Pub Med* or some other respectable data searcher can provide you with a reference list that earlier would have required weeks or more to acquire. Of course you still have to obtain and read the important papers—the computer provides no shortcut to this step.

If your prior experience has not taught you to use medical/scientific search engines your first efforts should consist of learning to use available resources. With this capability you can assemble a respectable body of background information on the subject you intend to investigate. General-purpose systems (Google, Yahoo) may give you useful information and are worth looking at. The National Library of Medicine *Pub Med* web site will provide the best overall medical/scientific search capability and is quite user friendly. Most of the papers which it identifies will have an attached abstract which at the least should show you whether the original is worth obtaining as a reference.

Among the services uniquely available at Western Michigan University School of Medicine, *Up-to-Date* produces a current, authoritative and well-referenced monograph on most general subjects of interest. It is a good place to start, but by itself will not yield a review of most subjects adequate to legitimize a research proposal. *MD Consult* surveys a database which is more limited than that accessible in *Pub Med* but has the advantage that many recent papers include a full text version, often in pdf format.

Additional resources for literature searching exist in limited, specialized fields; faculty mentors working in those fields can often direct you to these. Presentations at medical meetings will occasionally provide a preview of work not yet published, or perhaps work of marginal merit that the authors (or the journals) choose not to publish. Scanning abstracts from such meetings can broaden your bank of information on ideas proposed and work attempted.

Let's suppose that you have decided that you are truly interested in potential auto-borne allergens and want to see if others have published work in this field. Questions that you want to answer in the course of your literature survey might include:

- What do we know about techniques for environmental sampling for allergens?
- What about the relation between sampled levels and sensitization or production of allergic symptoms?
- Does sampling in a motor vehicle require adaptation of methods used out of doors or in a building?

- Would sampling produce different results in a stationary or moving vehicle?
- When a sample is obtained, how is allergen level measured and who is capable of providing reliable assay service?
- Is there prior literature on allergen exposure associated with riding in a motor vehicle?
- If earlier studies have been done, what geographic area was involved and what allergens were found—or looked for and not found?
- What has been the source of the allergen detected in the vehicle—outside allergen taken into the car vs. allergen arising from the car itself, its occupants or its litter?
- What effect, if any, does riding in a motor vehicle have on allergic symptoms?
- What about presence of pets in automobiles?

Remember that questions can go on without limit but you must focus and limit the scope of the investigation you ultimately undertake.

If you choose to search with *Pub Med* you will need a strategy and terms to implement the strategy. As an example your strategy may consist of varying combinations of terms which seem relevant:

Allergen, Allergy	Exposure, environment, location
Sampling	Automobile, Interior
Sensitization	Provocation
Asthma, Rhinitis	Rhinosinusitis, conjunctivitis

When you feel you have a thorough sampling of background information you should put together a portfolio which organizes and summarizes your findings. This forces you to integrate your thinking, providing a sound basis for the research proposal to follow. A well-written portfolio can serve as a powerful argument in favor of your project when it is reviewed by the Western Michigan University School of Medicine Research Department, the local Institutional Review Board and bodies whom you may approach for grant support. Looking ahead, this document can also provide an introduction and rationale for the protocol covering the proposed study and, probably with some modification, serve a similar purpose for a manuscript reporting the results of the research. This will take some time, may need revision, and should be in good form before it is exposed to any outside scrutiny.

Research Hypothesis

Based on your original ideas as modified by the results of the literature search you should now create a hypothesis.

The hypothesis should be:

- Simple
- Direct
- Testable

Don't allow yourself to be distracted by diversions such as "wouldn't it be nice to…", or "as long as we're doing the study why not…"

Specifically, with the concept of allergen exposure in an automobile, you might hypothesize that since house dust mites feed on human epidermal detritus they might find sustenance in auto upholstery. Thus you will try to devise a scheme for sampling auto interiors for mite allergen. Realizing that mites may not survive the cold of a Midwestern winter, you might want to sample autos in a southern state where there would be no exposure to freezing temperatures. Perhaps you could compare these results with samples from northern vehicles taken at the end of the summer season. Other qualifying features might develop after a thorough literature search has been accomplished.

One might ask a host of other somewhat related questions. What about animal dander? Is there residual outdoor allergen trapped in the auto interior? How does allergen recovered from auto upholstery or carpet relate to airborne allergen? What about food or mold allergens in the auto interior? These all sound like credible questions but all relate only indirectly to our interest in possible presence of mite allergen. Good research requires creativity but can get hamstrung if the creativity is uncontrolled.

Time required for this is variable but can easily be a "spare time" activity. You can think about your research hypothesis while you eat your lunch or drive to work.

Research Design

The research design should be appropriate for testing the hypothesis. This will take time and thought. General questions relating to a clinical study start with the hypothesis to be tested include the following:

- What study population will the study include?
- What features will exclude potential participants?
- How many study subjects will participate?
- What risks (or benefits) will participants incur?
- Are there privacy concerns?
- Informed consent—subject, parent(s), both?
- Where will the study take place? Who will do the hands-on work?
- Type and source of specimens, collected how and by whom.
- Specific measurements to be made and by whom.
- What is the time frame for the study?
- How will the data be analyzed?

While considering this plan you will want to consult with a statistician regarding study design. Of special importance will be estimates of sample size, and plans for data handling and analysis.

Specifically, for the study suggested above, elements of the research plan might include:

- Monograph providing background information and rationale for the study.
- (Hypothesis) Clinically significant amounts of mite allergen can be recovered from upholstery (and carpets?) in auto interiors. (How much allergen constitutes a "clinically significant" dose depends on findings from the literature search.)
- Vehicles suitable for sampling must be at least 3(?) years old with an odometer reading of at least 30,000 miles. Include new vehicles as controls?
- Vehicle must have fabric upholstery. Exclude if leather or vinyl seating or seat covers.
- Number of vehicles to be sampled to be determined.
- Selection of vehicles to be sampled regarding area of origin; also other inclusion and exclusion criteria.
- Any particular history regards vehicle type, age, use, etc? Will there be privacy issues concerning cars or owners?
- Specify sampling procedure.
- Handling/processing of sample.
- Assay procedure. Assay provider.
- Data analysis.

The research plan at this stage should be in written form, amenable to revision. This is not a final protocol.

Submit For Peer Review

We encourage peer review as a sit-down, face-to-face discussion activity. We do not view this as an inherently adversarial exercise but it should be open, frank and occasionally confrontational. The ultimate goal of all involved should be sound and ethical research design. This is an important and constructive part of the overall process.

For a resident-initiated project the peer review group might include:

- Faculty person(s) with the most expertise in the pertinent field
- Other faculty with relevant clinical or research experience
- Two senior residents
- Statistical consultant
- Others who may be able to contribute

Six to ten active participants work most efficiently. The resident-researcher should have primary responsibility for selecting the peer group. All participants should have the study plan and familiarize themselves with it prior to the meeting. They may need major supporting documents as well.

Issues to be addressed at the meeting include:

- Background information. Does the available information support the novelty and validity of the proposed project? Is any committee member aware of pertinent literature which the researcher has not considered and should? Will the proposed research have practical application? Do any in the peer group have personal experience which might benefit this effort?
- Study design. Is there any fundamental fallacy with the research hypothesis or design? Can patient and material resources within the institution support this effort? Can the research as described be carried out? Is the design practical and workable? Can it be simplified? Can committee members suggest better alternative approaches?

- Statistical considerations. Sample size? What factors will influence sample size determination? Plans for analysis? Are there design fallacies from the statistician's perspective?
- Patient and privacy matters. Are study demands and anticipated risk acceptable? Are plans for volunteer privacy protection adequate? Responsibility in case of adverse experiences.
- Funding. Suggestions on possible sources and how best to approach them.
- Anticipated problems. Administrative, clinical, scientific, ethical.

The document which results implies that all who contributed agree with important features of the study plan.

Write the Protocol

The following format is recommended when developing a research protocol:

- Title of the Study
- Names of all the Investigators
- Scientific Background
- Rationale
- Objectives
- Study Design
- Materials and Methods
- Statistical Analysis
- Expected Results
- Proposed Budget
- Bibliography
- Data Collection sheet
- Appendix: IRB Consent Forms (if necessary), device procedure manual, information from drug companies, etc.

When developing a protocol, all above bulleted guidelines (including statistical analysis) must be written prior to Clinical Research Department submission. Researchers should meet with the statistician, if needed, to develop the planned analysis.

Budget development and funding should be completed prior to protocol submission. The Director of Accounting is available for budget related questions.

Information technology needs and funding should be completed prior to protocol submission. The Director of Information Technology is available to discuss these needs and answer questions.

Personnel needs must be discussed with Human Resources. Anyone who is hired or volunteers to assist with your study must attend an orientation session within the Institution.

Basic Elements for Informed Consent Documents

Unless otherwise authorized by an IRB, research investigators must provide the following information to each subject in writing:

To enhance comprehension and readability, investigators are strongly urged to use a format in the body of the consent form that presents information in sections, introduced by headings, and that clearly and simply identifies and describes each of the elements to be discussed.

- A statement that the study involves research
- An explanation of the purpose of the research and the expected duration of the subject's participation
- A description of the procedures to be followed and identification of any procedures that are experimental
- A description of any foreseeable risks or discomforts to the subject, an estimate of their likelihood, and a description of what steps will be taken to prevent or minimize them
- A description of any benefits to the subject or to others that may reasonably be expected from the research. Monetary compensation is not a benefit. If compensation is to be provided to research subjects or healthy volunteers, the amount should be stated in the consent document
- A disclosure of any appropriate alternative procedures or courses of treatment that might be advantageous to the subject
- A statement describing to what extent records will be kept confidential, including a description of who may have access to research records

- For research involving more than minimal risk, an explanation and description of any compensation and any medical treatments that are available if research subjects are injured; where further information may be obtained, and whom to contact in the event of a research-related injury
- An explanation of whom to contact for answers to pertinent questions about the research and the research subject's rights (include the Clinical Center's Patient Representative and telephone number)
- A statement that participation is voluntary and that refusal to participate or discontinuing participation at any time will involve no penalty or loss of benefits to which the subject is otherwise entitled

RESEARCH PROJECT APPROVAL

Review by Western Michigan University School of Medicine Clinical Research Department

All studies conducted within Western Michigan University School of Medicine or carried out by Western Michigan University School of Medicine personnel, residents or medical students require an in-house review by the Western Michigan University School of Medicine Clinical Research Department. This review serves at least three purposes. First it notifies the Research Department that a new research project is planned within WMed. The Department maintains records of all studies active in the institution to assure compliance with federal regulations. The department is charged with auditing their progress periodically. Because of this all studies of any type carried out within Western Michigan University School of Medicine or by Western Michigan University School of Medicine personnel must be entered into their inventory and undergo review at this level.

The Clinical Research Committee review may also serve in lieu of peer review for departments within Western Michigan University School of Medicine that do not use a face-to-face meeting. Here the purpose of the review is to critique the scientific rationale and study design.

Finally the Clinical Research Department will consider matters of safety, ethics and privacy. An IRB will also consider these matters but the review within Western Michigan University School of Medicine may anticipate later questions and expedite the formal IRB review.

Protocol submission forms can be found on the Western Michigan University School of Medicine intranet. In addition, the Clinical Research Department could help in directly obtaining this form.

Note:

- All resident/student projects and case reports **MUST have a faculty sponsor**
- A binder for all study related materials should be maintained by the principal investigator and is subject to audit by the Western Michigan University School of Medicine Clinical Research Department

Institutional Review Board (IRB)

Any study which involves human subjects requires formal Institutional Review Board (IRB) review. The Bronson and Borgess IRBs, which we use most commonly, primarily concern themselves with safety and ethics.

Most IRBs meet once a month. Be aware of submission dates and meeting schedules. In addition to the protocol and directly supporting documents, these submissions will require a variety of administrative materials such as CV's, financial disclosures, privacy training documentation and more. Most of the forms will be available online and the IRB will advise you of their specific requirements.

For some studies "expedited" review might suffice. This could include minimal risk projects which represent minor modifications of previously approved studies or studies which involve minimal or no direct patient contact or manipulation. The chairman of the IRB will determine which studies qualify for expedited review.

Borgess IRB

- Studies involving patients or data obtained from Borgess Medical Center or its affiliates must be reviewed and approved by Borgess IRB: https://www.borgess.com/?pId=404.
- You must also obtain a HIPAA waiver from the IRB in order to view patient data at Borgess and/or its affiliates.
- Borgess IRB accepts the NIH research certification.

Bronson IRB

- Studies involving patients or data obtained from Bronson Methodist Hospital or its affiliates must be reviewed and approved by Bronson IRB: http://www.bronsonhealth.com/Research/BronsonIRB/page3899.html.html
- Bronson IRB accepts only the CITI research certification

If you will be collecting data from both institutions, you must have your protocol approved by both Borgess and Bronson IRBs.

Privacy Board

Some protocols may not need IRB review. These may involve chart reviews from Western Michigan University School of Medicine Clinic records in which information identifying specific individuals can be removed from the data base. In this case, review by the Clinical Research Department documents that these aspects have been considered and the protocol is acceptable for approval by the Privacy Board (PB).

Each institution Privacy Board is different but in general the PB will review study proposals that do not include the collection of protected health information (PHI). Consult with the Clinical Research Department concerning the suitability of your project for Privacy Board review will be the most appropriate path to follow.

The PB is not a substitute to the IRB. The PB may waive individual authorization for research that is not covered by the Common Rule if it determines that: it is a minimal risk to the privacy of individuals, that the research could not be conducted without the waiver or alteration, and that the research could not practically be conducted without access to the use of PHI.

The Privacy Board waiver application can be found in our institution on the intranet.

FUNDING

Identify a Source of Funding

Most research will require some money for materials, services, patient and personnel costs, etc. Obtaining funding requires some creativity. While the major source of research funds in academic medicine has long been the NIH, competition for the available pool of money is fierce. A first-time researcher should look to other sources.

Some pharmaceutical companies have made small grants for independent research, especially in fields which reflect their own research emphases. Western Michigan University School of Medicine researchers have also obtained money from other private sources (Blue Cross, private foundations).

Potential sources of funding will want to see a completed, IRB-reviewed study plan before they will review an application for support. Again this process will take time. The time from application to availability of funds may amount to several months. resent and Publish

Authorship Guidelines

Discuss Order of Authorship Early in The Research Process!

Who Should Be Included as an Author?

The decision of who to include as an author can sometimes be difficult. We suggest using the following guidelines when deciding authorship.

Authorship should include individuals who have:

- Made a significant contribution to the conception and design of the study
- Made an essential contribution in the actual accrual or analysis of data
- Participated in drafting the article or reviewing and/or revising it for content

Order of Authors

First Author	Leads the study and makes a major contribution to the work
Second Author	Co-investigator for the study, second only to the first author in terms of contribution to the study
Middle Author(s)	List in order of importance to the study
Last Author	The ringleader, the keeper of the keys, the mentor

Who Should be Acknowledged?

Those who do not meet the criteria listed above should be acknowledged. This includes people who provide: funds, technical services, materials, statistical analysis, etc.

Writing an Abstract

What is an Abstract? - An abstract is a short overview of your entire study. You may be using it as a submission for a meeting or as the summary for your manuscript. It should state ***WHAT*** you did, ***WHY*** you did it, ***HOW*** you did it, ***WHAT*** you found, and ***WHAT*** it means. Abstracts that are well written will make the reader want to learn more about the research.

Drafting Your Abstract - Before you begin, review the meeting or journal abstract guidelines for specific criteria (e.g., margins, word/page limit, font size/style, headings). Next, start by writing one or two sentences that summarize each section of the abstract. **Be concise**--say only what is essential, using no more words than necessary to convey meaning.

The basic components of most abstracts are:

Introduction/Study Objective

- What are the specific aims for this study?
- Why is this project interesting or important?

Methods

- If this is a clinical study, describe your patients, including brief inclusion/exclusion criteria
- Briefly explain your procedures
- Define the primary outcome variable
- If statistical tests were run, define your criterion for significance (e.g., $p < 0.05$)

Results

- What were the major findings of your study?

Discussion/Conclusions

- Summarize the major findings
- If you have space, briefly discuss your results relative to current findings in the literature
- The last one or two lines of the abstract should be the big finish.

Throughout the abstract drafting process, ask your mentor and all other co-authors to review the abstract and provide you with feedback. For your final draft, make sure the abstract "flows" logically by adding more descriptive information and transitional sentences. (See Appendix for abstract examples)

Creating a Poster

General - Each presentation should include an introduction to the topic, key points about the topic, and a summary of the results or key points. Do not try to present details at length on a poster; instead, be prepared to discuss the details with your viewers.

Your poster should be self-explanatory. This is helpful for people who view it when you are not present, and it frees you when you are present to supplement and discuss particular points raised by an inquiry. The poster session offers a more intimate forum for discussions than an oral presentation, but this becomes more difficult if you are obligated to devote most of your time to merely explaining your poster to a succession of viewers.

Type Size, Graphics - Unless you are a licensed calligrapher, use a computer to produce crisp, professional-looking type and graphics. Your poster will be viewed from a distance (3' or more). Your "Title and Author" section should be in lettering at least 1" high. All other lettering should be at least 3/8" high. Charts, drawings, and illustrations should be similar to those used in making slides (i.e., simple and heavily drawn). Use a heavy, legible font that is free from unnecessary ornamentation (such as Arial). Use a laser printer, if possible. "Landscape" formatting of pages can increase line length, thereby enhancing readability.

Illustrations, Photographs, and Drawings - Omit unnecessary detail and ornate, gratuitous graphics. Tables of raw data are NOT informative or appealing as graphs, and the numbers are not remembered when your viewers walk away. Save such archival information for handouts. Provide each figure with a legend stating a clear, concise message in large type - at least 3/8" high. If necessary, detailed information can be provided in smaller type below.

Arrangement, Content - The poster platforms for Research Day measure six feet in height (top to floor) by four feet in width.

The title and author name(s) (in lettering at least 1" high) should be centered at the top of the platform. Consistency will make it easier for viewers to scan and browse the many posters in the room. In addition, you should include the author affiliation(s) in smaller type (but not less than 3/8") directly below the name(s).

The human, English-reading eye moves from left to right. In general, lay out your poster so that the information flows from left to right rather than in vertical columns. Your introduction should be placed at the upper left and your conclusion to the lower right. Number each part of the poster so that the flow of information will be clear to all. Adding arrows to the panels also helps to indicate the flow.

Sample Poster Arrangement - Below is a sample poster arrangement for a clinical study:

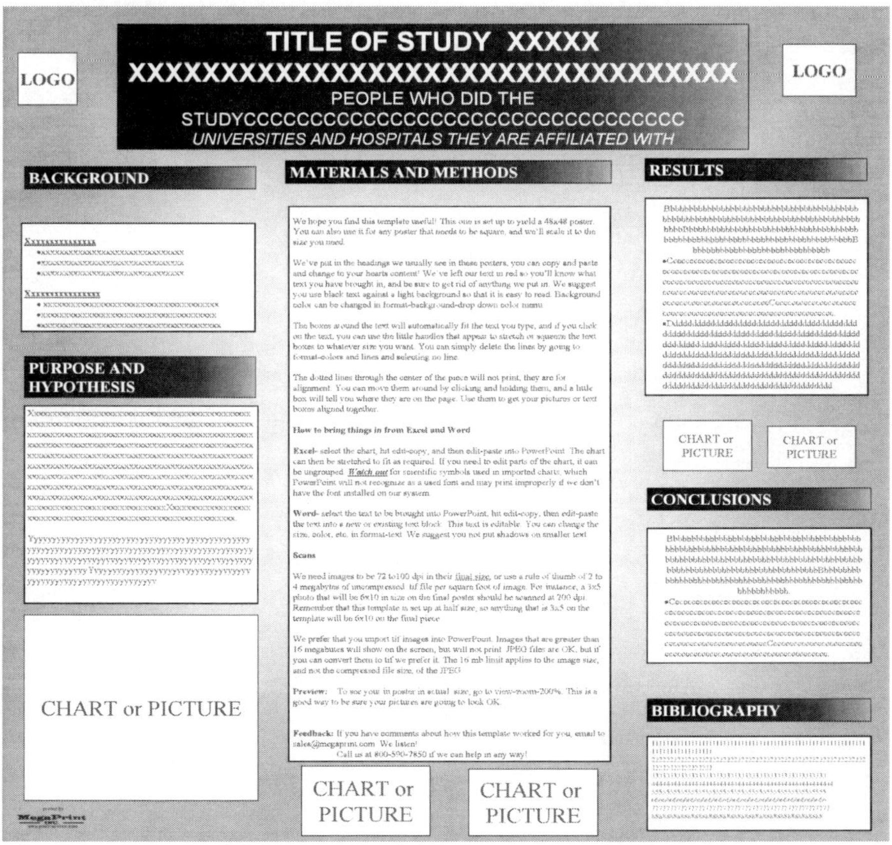

Creating a Powerpoint

Number of Slides - Your first tendency may be to treat this like the lightning round, flashing 30 slides a second. This strobe light effect can cause seizures and is widely regarded as bad form. A good rule of thumb is to show one or two slides per minute, recognizing that extra time may be needed to orient your audience to slides displaying data.

Color - Make sure your slides consist of contrasting colors that will show up in a darkened room. Beware of the overly bright colors as well as overly distracting background patterns.

Slide Format –

- For text slides, use a larger font; think 28 to 40 point, as opposed to 12 point
- No more than four or five bullets per slide; resist the temptation to put everything you're going to say on the slide
- Data slides with a two-column table should have no more than five rows; three-column tables should have no more than three rows

Presentation

Title slide (1 slide)

- The title in a magnificent, oversize font
- All of the authors (tip – always include the middle initial for each author)
- All of the institutions (this includes the institutional affiliations for the authors as well as the institution where the research was conducted)
- If a resident is involved, Western Michigan University School of Medicine should ALWAYS be listed
- If a MSU medical student is involved, MSU-CHM should ALWAYS be listed

Significance/Background/Specific Aims (2-3 slides)

- Appropriate attention getter
- Rationale for study
- Study questions/hypotheses

Methods (2-4 slides)

- Design
- Sampling
- Data collection
- Key variables
- Definitions
- Sample size/statistics

Results (4-5 slides)

- First choice for results presentation is a **Figure**
- Second choice: **Table**
- Third choice: **Text**
- Don't over cram any of the above choices
- If you absolutely need to include an overly complex **Figure**, **Table** or **Algorithm**, please provide a handout to your audience as support material
- Highlight your most interesting results

Discussion (2-4 slides) - Discuss your results, relative to the current literature

Conclusion (1 slide) - The big finish. No matter how weak your data, always include a conclusions slide

Acknowledgments (1 slide) - List of organization(s) funding the project. Thank you to any and all persons who helped with the study, but do not fit author criteria

Preparing a Manuscript

Where to Start - Ask your faculty mentor for a list of journals suitable for your manuscript. Review those journals to see the types of articles they publish.

Submission Guidelines - Once you have chosen an appropriate journal, make sure to review the author guidelines for submission ***before*** you begin writing your article. http://mulford.meduohio.edu/instr/ links to over 3000 journals and their instructions for authors. It is also useful to obtain a sample article from the selected journal and review the style and flow in one of their manuscripts.

Authoring/Proofreading/Reviewing Your Article - For every manuscript, there is usually one author who has the primary responsibility for writing the first draft.

> ***When complete, distribute the first draft to all co-authors so everyone can participate in the authoring/drafting process.***

This cycle of writing/revision is continued for each version of the draft. The next-to-last draft of the manuscript should be distributed to the following for proofreading and editing:

- Residency Program or Research Department Director
- Western Michigan University School of Medicine Clinical Research Department

Comments should then be reviewed by all of the authors and used for the preparation of the finalized form of the manuscript. You should now be ready to submit.

Case Report/Series Outline

Instructions for creating the basic narrative used to describe a case study (1- 5 patients) When writing up your report refrain from using identifying data, such as date of birth, date of service, patient name/initials or medical record number. Do not use case when referring to a person - a case is an instance of disease, a patient is a person.

Title - Descriptive title of the case report/series; keep it tight, no 100 word titles.

Introduction - The introduction should be brief; tell why the case is important and why it is being reported. Case studies usually respond to one of the following generic topics but use specific information from the case being presented.

- An unexpected association between diseases or symptoms
- An unexpected event in the course of observing or treating a patient
- Findings that shed new light on the possible pathogenesis of a disease or an adverse effect
- Unique or rare features of a disease
- Unique therapeutic approaches

Significance/Uniqueness of Case - Using the literature, establish any previous work that is related to your research question. Make clear to your reader whether this is the first instance of this case ever reported, or how many have been reported previously. The essential characteristic of a publishable case report is educational value. After all, nobody is going to change the way they practice medicine based upon one case report. In addition, it is not true that a report must tell of a unique finding. Some case reports are published because they support the findings in previously published cases or because they are useful reminders of an important point in diagnosis or treatment.

Patient Description - Describe the patient, including: gender, age, BMI, morbidities, use of illegal substances and medications, notable results of exams and tests, and differential diagnosis or diagnoses considered. Think about the patient information you would like to know as background information and provide it in this section. Give all of the basics and add the specifics pertinent to the case.

Therapeutic Intervention

Describe all therapeutic interventions conducted during the course of treatment. Only provide the results of relevant examinations and laboratory tests. List the laboratory's ranges of normal values for any unusual tests performed.

Response to Treatment - Describe the outcome of treatment including final diagnosis.

Discussion - The purpose of the discussion is to explain anything that isn't clear in the case description and to offer interpretations of findings. It's also the place to indicate why the intervention used for your case was different from similar cases reported previously. Make clear any important point that isn't explained in the case descriptions. For example, if you reported that liver enzymes were elevated but no significant liver dysfunction was found, tell the reader in the discussion section why the enzymes were elevated. Also discuss implications for the field.

Conclusions - This should be brief, three sentences tops. If you're at a loss for words, you can either do a combined discussion/conclusions section, or just have a conclusions section that reiterates the importance of your case.

Other Requirements

1) Single case reports do not require IRB approval. Two or more case reports would need IRB consideration even though they are generally exempted.
2) If you are using a photo with identifying features (e.g., face, tattoo, birthmark), you must have written approval from the patient.

Clinical/Basic Science Study Outline

Instructions for Creating the Basic Narrative Used to Describe Your Study

Title - Descriptive title of the research project; keep it tight, no 100 word titles.

Research Question - Specify the specific aims for your study.

Significance - Using the literature, establish any previous work related to your research question. This section should describe the gaping hole in the literature and how your specific aims will attempt to address it.

Methods - The next four sections encompass the methods. Traditionally, this grouping has been headed "Methods" or "Materials and Methods" but studies involving human subjects usually label this section "Patients and Methods".

Design - What research design was used to address your specific aims? Examples include case series, case-control, retrospective cohort, cross-sectional, prospective cohort and randomized controlled trial. (The description "retrospective chart review" is not a study design. Instead, consider using "case series" or "retrospective cohort study.")

Subjects - This is where you would include your patient information but, not all studies involve patients so adjust your heading accordingly. For example, you could have done an animal study, worked with cells or even run a meta-analysis. Assuming this is a clinical study, however, you need to provide information to your reader concerning your subjects. You should describe where you obtained your subjects, over what time period and the specific inclusion and exclusion criteria used. If this was a prospective study you will need to state whether informed consent was obtained.

Procedures/Variables/Definitions - This section basically describes your experimental treatments/interventions (if any), your methods of obtaining your data and a description of your variables. Likewise, you would provide information about a chart review in this section as well. Provide information about your primary outcome variable, as well as all secondary outcome variables. At times it will be necessary to define these variables, so be precise.

Analyses - - Use this section to provide a thorough description of the statistical tests used, your sample size justification (if pertinent to your study) and your criterion for significance (e.g., $P < 0.05$).

Results - Here's where you provide the results from your study. Make frequent and liberal use of tables and figures. Make sure that the reader is very aware of what you consider to be the major findings from your study. This is also a place to remark upon some of the minor findings that did not make their way into any of your tables and figures.

Discussion - The discussion section is used to summarize the findings from your study and to

interpret your results relative to current findings in the literature.

Conclusions - - This should be brief, three sentences tops. If you're at a loss for words, you can either do a combined discussion/conclusions section or just have a conclusions section that reiterates the importance of your study.

Kalamazoo Community Medical and Health Sciences Research Day

For over 30 years, the Kalamazoo Community Medical and Health Sciences have sponsored an annual Research Day. This special forum provides an opportunity for faculty, residents, medical students, health professional students, to present the latest findings from their research studies.

The emphasis of Research Day is educational - allowing researchers an opportunity to present their work in a supportive, constructive learning environment. All presentations are critiqued by judges, with feedback immediately available to all presenters. This is especially useful for investigators who are using this event to practice and refine their presentations prior to delivery at a regional or national conference.

Research Day also provides an opportunity to meet and discuss projects with other researchers and to survey the breadth of area research interests.

We invite you to support and participate in Research Day every year.

For further details about Western Michigan University School of Medicine Research Day, visit the following web link: http://med.wmich.edu/node/1.

ACKNOWLEDGMENTS

We would like to thank the following contributors to this Brief "Guide to Research":

Dr. Carter Brooks, from our institution.

Grand Rapids Medical Education and Research Center; in particular Dr. Alan Davis, Dr. Tom Summerfelt, Linda Youmans and Tracy Frieswyk.

Michigan State University–College of Human Medicine Research Guidelines.

Drs. Matthew Bollier, Todd Ream, Gregory Hodgman, Luis H. Toledo-Pereyra, Craig Kaml, Kieran Fogarty, Christina Preusz, William Fales and Fernando Lopez-Neblina for allowing us to use their abstracts on this Guide.

APPENDIX A - EXAMPLE OF A CASE REPORT ABSTRACT

Matthew Bollier[1], Todd Ream[2] and Gregory Hodgman[3]

[1]Michigan State University- Kalamazoo Center for Medical Studies, Kalamazoo, MI, US

[2]Kalamazoo Orthopaedic Clinic; Kalamazoo, MI, US

[3]Bronson Advanced Radiology, Kalamazoo, MI, US

Isolated Popliteus Muscle Rupture with Neurovascular Compression Requiring Surgical Decompression

OBJECTIVE: We report the unique case of an isolated popliteus muscle rupture that led to compression of the posterior tibial nerve and vein in the popliteal fossa requiring surgical decompression. There have been three case reports of a popliteus muscle injury causing posterior tibial nerve palsy, but surgical decompression of this problem has not been previously described. This interesting case demonstrates the anatomy of the posterior aspect of the knee, highlights the importance of a thorough physical exam and advanced imaging techniques, and reviews the current literature on neurovascular compression after a popliteus muscle injury.

METHODS: A 34 year-old man presented to the emergency room with severe proximal posterolateral calf pain and swelling, knee effusion, plantar foot dysesthesias, and weakness of great toe plantarflexion after an external rotation injury to his knee two weeks prior while on duty as a police officer. Lower extremity ultrasound demonstrated multiple calf deep vein thrombosis. MRI with gadolinium revealed a non-enhancing popliteus muscle consistent with muscle necrosis. It also revealed extensive surrounding edema and hemorrhage compressing the posterior tibial nerve and vein against the fibrous soleus arch. The patient demonstrated worsening posterolateral calf pain, progressive toe flexion weakness (0/5), ankle plantarflexion weakness (1/5), and decreased plantar foot sensation. Using a posterior approach to the knee, urgent surgical decompression of the posterior tibial nerve was performed by releasing the fibrous soleus arch. Necrotic appearing popliteus muscle was excised.

RESULTS: The patient's pain resolved immediately after decompression. Lower extremity ultrasound demonstrated resolution of this deep vein thrombosis after decompression. He returned to work 2 months after surgery. At nine months post-operatively, ankle plantarflexion strength was 5/5 and great toe plantar flexion was 1/5. Although improved, sensation is still decreased on the plantar aspect of the foot.

CONCLUSION: An isolated popliteus muscle rupture from a knee external rotation injury and subsequent necrosis caused an inflammatory mass effect in the popliteal fossa compressing the posterior tibial nerve and vein against the soleus arch. This condition must be considered when a patient presents with proximal calf pain, tenderness, and swelling. In this case, surgical decompression relieved the intense neuropathic pain and allowed partial posterior tibial nerve recovery.

Appendix B - Example of Medical Humanities Abstract

Luis H. Toledo-Pereyra[1], *Craig A. Kaml*[2] *and Kieran Fogarty*[2]
[1] Western Michigan University School of Medicine,
Michigan State University College of Human Medicine,
Michigan State University College of Osteopathic Medicine,
Kalamazoo, MI, US
[2]Departments of Research and Surgery, Michigan State University,
Kalamazoo Center for Medical Studies, Borgess Research Institute
and Western Michigan University, Kalamazoo, MI, US

Teaching Medicine through the History of Disease: An Innovative Approach to Medical Education

BACKGROUND: Current teaching methods to educate medical students are based on scientific principles of medicine. Little or no attention has been paid to utilizing medical humanities as a mean to improve student knowledge and retention.

OBJECTIVES: The aims of this project were to: 1. promote learning among medical students by adopting a blended approach of synchronous and asynchronous modalities; 2. create international learning communities involving American and Mexican universities; 3. design, implement and evaluate an information system that includes a synchronous distance learning platform, a knowledge management system and an interactive historical timeline and; 4. assess and evaluate the effectiveness of both the history of disease synchronous class meetings and the asynchronous component of the information system.

MATERIAL AND METHODS: The student population consisted of 87 to 168 medical students and pre-med undergraduate students who participated in any of five learning modules offered in the curriculum. The content of the lecture series was formulated to progressively expose medical students to the historical path of discovery, research and the current understanding of Alzheimer's disease. Lecture 1 dealt with "History of Neuroscience and Dementia"; Lecture 2 presented "Dr. Alois Alzheimer: His Life and Work"; Lecture 3 introduced "Historic Profile of Alzheimer Disease"; Lecture 4, analyzed "Modern Concepts of

Alzheimer's Disease"; and Lecture 5 discussed "Alzheimer Disease: Treatment and Prevention".

Participants were spread across three time zones and six universities. Institutions included Michigan State University (MSU) at East Lansing and Kalamazoo, University of Illinois-Chicago, Western Michigan University-Kalamazoo and University of Nuevo-Mexico. The subjects were successful in navigating the on-line curriculum from any location and participation in pre/post assessments. The identified confounding variables of interest were gender, student status, practice interest, location of the medical school or university (domestic or international) and most importantly results of the self-administered pre and post lecture testing questionnaires. Statistical Analysis included student's t-test and analysis of variance when applicable. Mean and standard deviation of the mean were used. Significance was reached at $p \leq 0.05$.

RESULTS: There were no significant differences in gender, student status, or practice interest except for lecture 3; and location except for lectures 1 and 2. A significant difference in pre- and post-test examination was noted in all lectures except lecture 4 even though the mean was clearly increased after testing.

CONCLUSION: This study statistically supported that the students were able to increase their knowledge and score testing after the delivery of the curriculum above discussed. Thus, teaching through the history of disease is a viable, innovative and worthwhile platform to learn medicine in a more effective and substantial way.

This study was supported by NIH and lasted five years from conception to completion.

APPENDIX C - EXAMPLE OF BASIC SCIENCES ABSTRACT

Fernando López-Neblina[1] and Luis H. Toledo-Pereyra[1,2]

[1]Universidad Autonoma de Baja California, Department of Research, Laboratory of Experimental Medicine, Mexicali, Baja California, Mexico,

[2] Western Michigan University School of Medicine,
Michigan State University College of Human Medicine,
Michigan State University College of Osteopathic Medicine,
Kalamazoo, MI, US

Ryanodine Receptor Antagonist Modulates the Expression of Hsp70 in Hepatic Ischemia and Reperfusion

BACKGROUND: Heat shock proteins (Hsps) are ubiquitously expressed and highly conserved families of molecules. Their immune reactivity has been implicated in the pathogenesis of inflammatory conditions such as autoimmune and cardiovascular diseases. Hsps under physiological conditions act as molecular chaperones. Hsps overexpression has been observed *in vivo* and *in vitro* under stresses including heat, nutrient deprivation and ischemia.

Dantrolene is a ryanodine receptor (RyR) antagonist. The RyR Ca^{++} release channel mobilizes Ca^{++} from internal calcium stores to support a variety of cellular functions, including inflammatory pathways. We hypothesized that dantrolene, due to its internal Ca^{++} release inhibitory effect, could exert a protective effect in liver ischemia and reperfusion (I/R) through the increment on the expression of Hsp70.

MATERIAL AND METHODS: Mice subjected to 90 minutes of partial (70-80%) hepatic ischemia and three hours of reperfusion were divided into five groups (n=5/group): Sham, Ischemic Control, and the Dantrolene 1mg/kg group which was studied at three different times of administration: 15 minutes before reperfusion (DAN-PRE), at the time of reperfusion (DAN-@RP) and 15 minutes after reperfusion (DAN-POST). The parameters measured at three hours of reperfusion included liver function tests (ALT and AST), histological assessment and Hsp70 measurements. Hsp70 was measured in liver homogenates by ELISA. Histopathology was carefully analyzed using the Suzuki classification for ischemic damage. Statistical analysis included Analysis of Variance setting significance at p values < 0.05. Values were expressed as mean $\pm$ standard deviation (M $\pm$ SD).

RESULTS: It was demonstrated that the RyR antagonist dantrolene offered the most significant protection for the ischemic liver when given at the time of reperfusion. AST significantly differed between the control group and the group receiving 1mg/kg at the time of reperfusion (p=0.01). ALT showed a statistically significant decrease in the DAN-PRE treated group and a decrease, although not significant, in the DAN-@RP. Histological examination demonstrated a significant decrease in vacuolization in the DAN-PRE and DAN-@RP when compared to the IC (p<0.05). Necrosis was reduced only when dantrolene was used at the time of reperfusion. Hsp70 was significantly higher in the DAN-@RP (19.22 $\pm$ 5.0) when compared to ischemic control (9.33 $\pm$ 2.3), sham (6.71 $\pm$ 1.7) and DAN-PRE (9.84 $\pm$ 3.6) (p<0.05).

CONCLUSION: Dantrolene demonstrated a protective effect in liver I/R by blocking the release of internal Ca^{++} and increasing the expression of the protective chaperone protein Hsp70.

APPENDIX D - EXAMPLE OF CLINICAL STUDY ABSTRACT

Christina Preusz and William Fales
Emergency Medicine, Michigan State University/Kalamazoo Center for Medical Studies, Kalamazoo, MI, US

Impact of New Resuscitation Guidelines on Out-of-Hospital Cardiac Arrest Survival

OBJECTIVE: To measure the impact on survival from out-of-hospital cardiac arrest (OHCA) upon implementation of new resuscitation guidelines.

METHODS: This study occurred within a single, countywide EMS system serving a population of 240,536 (562 square miles). This was a cohort study of persons receiving OHCA resuscitation, comparing patients during a prospectively defined intervention period (March 1, 2006 to April 31, 2007) with those in a historical control period (January 1, 2005 to February 28, 2006). During the intervention period (IP) patients were treated based on new resuscitation guidelines. Protocols were changed to reflect increased emphasis on CPR, elimination of stacked shocks, immediate resumption of CPR after defibrillation, minimization of all interruptions in chest compressions, and a change to the Combitube™ as the primary advanced airway. EMS personnel received 2 hours of training in these changes. Patients during the control period (CP) were treated under the previous guidelines. The primary outcome was survival to hospital discharge. Data were collected and analyzed in a manner consistent with the Utstein model for CA reporting resulting in progressively defined subsets of cardiac arrest types. Analysis was conducted using SAS version 9.1 at 5% level of significance using t tests, χ^2 tests, or Fisher tests. Logistic regression was used to adjust for relevant covariates and adjusted ORs and 95% confidence intervals (CIs) were determined. Univariate comparisons were conducted to identify differences in distribution of covariates between periods with comparisons with $P<.20$ included for consideration in the final logistic regression model.

RESULTS: Resuscitations were initiated in 168 patients during CP and 172 patients during the IP. The CP and IP patients were similar in terms of age, gender, race, OHCA location type, percent bystander witness, percent receiving bystander CPR, and percent with automated defibrillator use. Paramedic response time was slightly slower during the CP than during the IP (mean minutes, 7.1 vs. 6.4; p=.0401). Post-arrest therapeutic hypothermia was used 14 times (8.1%) during the IP and not at all during the CP. Outcome data for all patients and for sub-groups are provided in the table below. The adjusted odds ratio using the linear regression model for survival to discharge for all attempted resuscitations was 3.74; 95% CI=2.52-5.55). In terms of discharge location, 5.4% of patients survived to be discharged home in the CP vs. 14.5% during the IP (p=.0024).

Table. Survival to Hospital Admission and Discharge

	Admitted				Discharged			
	CP % (n)	IP % (n)	p	OR (95% CI)	CP % (n)	IP % (n)	p	OR (95% CI)
All Resuscitations	24.0 (40)	36.6 (63)	0.0056	1.84 (1.41-2.94)	8.9 (15)	16.9 (29)	0.0147	2.07 (1.07-4.02)
Cardiac Etiology	24.4 (30)	38.8 (45)	0.0083	1.96 (1.13-3.43)	10.6 (13)	21.6 (25)	0.0102	2.32 (1.13-4.80)
CE + Bystander Witnessed	27.1 (19)	55.6 (35)	0.0005	3.36 (1.62-6.92)	10.0 (7)	33.3 (21)	0.0045	4.50 (1.76-11.52)
CE + BW + Initial Rhythm VF	38.7 (12)	70.5 (31)	0.0031	3.78 (1.43-9.96)	19.4 (6)	45.5 (20)	0.0097	3.47 1.19-10.13

Abbreviations: CP=control period, IP=intervention period, OR=odds ratio, CE=cardiac etiology, BW=bystander witnessed, VF=ventricular fibrillation.

CONCLUSION: Implementation of new resuscitation guidelines, including a change to the CombitubeTM as the primary advanced airway, was associated with improved hospital admission and survival to hospital discharge for OHCA patients within this EMS system. There was a significant improvement in the percent of patients who survived to be discharged to home after implementation of these new guidelines.

A Final Note of Appreciation

This Brief "Guide to Research" represents the works of various researchers, which we amalgamated and freely used to bring about the best of the research process. In this case, the works of Dr. Carter Brooks (Retired) from Pediatrics at our institution and Dr. Alan Davis, Dr. Tom Summerfelt, Linda Youmans and Tracy Frieswyk of the Grand Rapids Medical Education and Research Center were the individuals from whom we utilized their writings to complete this booklet. We identified the best portions of their works and presented them in an educational manner. We appreciate their contribution to bring about this work in progress. We also thank Dawn Chovanec, RN, Sandra Sheppard, RN, and Barbara Lupina from the Clinical Research Department of Western Michigan University School of Medicine for helping to compose and rearrange the works of the various research groups mentioned above. We look forward to your comments and ideas for improving research at Western Michigan University School of Medicine.

Luis H. Toledo-Pereyra

In: Principles of Research
Editor: Luis H. Toledo-Pereyra
ISBN: 978-1-62417-968-6

Appendix II

Western Michigan University School of Medicine (WMed) Research Protocol Submission Guidelines and Directions

Luis H. Toledo-Pereyra
Western Michigan University School of Medicine,
Michigan State University College of Human Medicine,
Michigan State University College of Osteopathic Medicine,
Kalamazoo, MI, US

I Obtain and utilize the Clinical Research Department Submission Guidelines and Directions for reference and submit the Submission Form with your protocol to the WMed Research Department. These are found on the WMed Intranet in the Research Section.

II Develop your protocol and include the items below.

  a The following format is recommended when developing a research protocol:

  - Title of the study
  - Names of all the Investigators
  - Scientific background (1 page)
  - Rationale (½ page)
  - Objectives (½ page)
  - Study Design (1 page)

- Materials and Methods (1 page)
- Statistical Analysis (½ page)
- Expected Results (½ page)
- Proposed Budget
- Bibliography
- Appendix: IRB Consent Forms (if necessary), device procedure manual, information from drug companies, etc.

b When developing a non-industry (academic, government, or private) sponsored research project, all above bulleted guidelines (including statistical analysis) *must be written prior to the Clinical Research Department submission.* Researchers should meet with the WMed statistician, if needed, to develop the planned analysis. Also, we recommend meeting with the Director of Clinical Research or the Clinical Research Coordinator.

c Budget development and funding should be completed prior to protocol submission. The WMed Director of Accounting is available for budget related questions.

d Information technology needs and funding should be completed prior to protocol submission. The WMed Director of Information Technology is available to discuss these needs and answer questions.

e For assistance with any of the above, please contact the WMed Director of Clinical Research or a Research Coordinator.

III Complete Human Participant Protection Education for Research is required of all investigators

For instructions online, go to the internet and use "clinicaltrials/learning/humanparticipant".

a This education is required of all personnel listed on the study. Protocol approval is based upon successful completion and submission of documentation of this education.

b The *NIH Human Participant Protection Education for Research* self study course is recommended. Takes approximately 1-2 hours, but you can sign in/sign out at your convenience.

c Print your certificate of completion for submission to the research department with the protocol.

d Completion of an education program concerning Human Participant Protection is also required to submit to both IRB hospitals in the community, the Bronson IRB and Borgess IRB. Bronson IRB requires the CITI (Collaborative Institutional Training Initiative) training program which can be obtained through the internet. Borgess IRB accepts the NIH Human Participant Protection Program.

IV Complete the WMed Privacy Rule (HIPAA) for Researchers Education

a This education is required of all personnel listed on the study. Protocol approval is based upon successful completion and submission of documentation of this education.

b After submission of your research study to the Research Department, you will be contacted by the WMed NetLearning Systems Administrator with access information to the *WMed Privacy Rule for Researchers* education.

c It takes approximately 15 minutes to complete this training.

d Once successfully completed with a minimum 80% pass rate, a certificate will be printed by the WMed NetLearning Systems Administrator and forwarded to the Clinical Research Department.

V Research Financial Conflict of Interest

a. Determine if a financial conflict of interest applies to each investigator on the study by reviewing the WMed policy of *Research Financial Conflict of Interest* and answering the questions on the *WMed Research Conflict of Interest Financial Disclosure Statement* form.

b. If no financial conflict exists, complete the appropriate check box. No further action required.

c. If a financial conflict or potential for a financial conflict exists, mark the appropriate check box. Submit, along with your protocol, the completed *WMed Research Conflict of Interest Financial Disclosure Statement* for every researcher where the conflict is identified. This form is located on the WMed Intranet: Research Department or solicit it directly from the Clinical Research office.

d. The Director of Clinical Research will determine if a Financial Conflict of Interest exists, and if it does, shall provide a copy of their conclusions and recommendations to address the Conflict of Interest to the Director of Compliance.

e. You will be notified of the decision and actions you are required to complete for the submission process.

f. The approval of your research study is contingent upon satisfactory resolution of all Financial Conflict of Interest concerns.

VI WMed Privacy Board Review

a The Privacy Board review is required for all studies that meet the following criteria:

- the use or disclosure of protected health or private information, not covered by an informed consent or assent, or,
- the research could not practically be conducted without the waiver or alteration or,
- the research could not practically be conducted without access to and use of the protected health or private information or,
- IRB approval is not required but the study includes privacy information.

b Complete and submit the *Request for Waiver of Authorization to Use and Disclose Protected Health Information for Research Purposes* form. This form is located on the WMed Intranet: Clinical Research Department.

VII Complete Submission Form.

VIII The following documents must be submitted to the WMed Clinical Research Department:

Documents	Number of Copies
Submission Form	2 copies
Protocol	4 copies
Informed Consent, if applicable	4 copies
Curriculum vitae, for all investigators	1 copy
Study Summary, for IRB submission	1 copy
Budget, if receiving funding from any source	1 copy
Certification of Completion of NIH *Human Participant Protections Education for Research* for each person listed on protocol	1 copy
Certification of Completion and quiz for *Privacy Rule (HIPAA) for Researchers* for each person listed on protocol	1 copy
Research Conflict of Interest Financial Disclosure Statement for each investigator – if applicable	1 copy
Contract/Letter of Agreement for Industry Sponsored or studies receiving grants with contracts	1 copy

IX A Study Summary is usually required if submitting to an IRB. Bronson and Borgess IRBs require a Study Summary. See the specific requirements of the IRB when developing your summary.

Sample Summary: Provide a brief statement for each of the following:

a Title of the project
b Principal Investigator and Co-Investigators
c Funding Source
d Purpose of Study
e Procedure of the Study:
  i Study design
  ii Summary of methods
f Subjects:
  iii Eligibility Criteria
  iv Method of Selection and Recruitment
g Potential Risks to the Subject
h Safety monitoring procedures
i Benefits:
  v Potential Benefits to the Subject
  vi Scientific Benefits

X Your protocol will be peer-reviewed by two members of the Clinical Research Committee.
a The following areas will be evaluated during the peer-review process:
- Clearly-stated hypothesis
- Expected significance of this work
- Experimental design and methods
- Medical utility in patient therapy, prevention or diagnosis
- Risk/Benefit Ratio
- Statistical Analysis
- Suitability of investigator to carry out this work

b Each topic will receive a score using the following scale:
4 = Exceeds Standards
2 = Need Improvement
3 = Meets Standards
1 = Unsatisfactory

c Scores of 3 or 4 will receive Clinical Research Committee approval once WMed Clinical Research Department impact is evaluated.

d For any scores of 1 or 2: Copies of all evaluations, without reviewer names, will be forwarded to the researcher. You **must** respond to the scores by making recommended changes and resubmit revised protocol for re-evaluation**.** The sooner you respond, the sooner you may start your research project (after IRB approval obtained.) DO NOT ignore this step. The Research

Committee's Peer Review process is designed to help you produce a quality, hopefully publishable project.

e The revised protocol and initial scores will be sent to the reviewer(s) that gave initial scores of 1 or 2. The reviewer(s) again are asked to return the evaluation forms within 5 days.

f Preliminary Clinical Research Committee approval based on scientific merit is granted if:

- All evaluations are satisfactory (3 or 4).
- Privacy Board review approval – if needed
- Human Participant Protection Education certificate of completion received or on file in the Research Department.
- HIPAA, Privacy Rule, certificate of education received or on file in the Research Department.
- Financial Conflict of Interest Statement documented.

g Final Clinical Research Committee approval is based on review and approval of the following WMed departments:

- Human Resources
- Accounting
- Information Technology
- Administration

XI WMed Department Reviews and Final Associate Dean for Faculty and Clinical Affairs Approval

a The department directors or their designee of human resources, accounting, and information technology review all protocols for impact of resources required to conduct the research.

b The principle investigator is responsible to obtain additional resources required for their research and must confirm acquisition of these provisions with the department directors.

c Human resources, accounting and information technology department directors sign off on research projects when all required resources have been identified and provided in order to conduct the research.

d Once department directors of human resources, accounting and information technology have signed off on the research project, the final review is conducted by the Associate Dean for Faculty and Clinical Affairs and approval given to proceed.

XII Industry sponsored or studies receiving grants with contracts and or letters of agreement:

a The Associate Dean for Faculty and Clinical Affairs and the Associate Dean for Finances are the only authorized signers of WMed contracts or letters of agreement.

b All contracts and/or letters of agreement must be signed by the CEO regardless of whether they also require the investigator to sign. Add a signature line for Dr. Burns, Associate Dean for Faculty and Clinical Affairs on the signature page of the Contract/Letter of Agreement.

c All funds are payable to WMed.

d Contracts or letters of agreement to conduct research at WMed must contain the following. Legal jargon may differ, but the intent must be clear. These contracts or letters of agreement must be reviewed and approved by the Associate Dean for Finances prior to submission to the Associate Dean for Faculty and Clinical Affairs for signatory approval. Included are:

1. **A hold harmless clause** – This clause may also be called an indemnification clause or letter. It states that we (WMed) are not liable for any acts by the company (the sponsor) that are outside the scope of our control. The sponsor also has the reciprocal right. Additionally, WMed is not liable during an industry sponsored clinical trial should there be a problem with a patient caused by the drugs themselves.
2. **A termination clause** – This clause permits us to cancel our participation in a study should WMed feel such a step was appropriate. The termination clause should include that WMed will still receive payment for whatever work has been done to date. In most contracts, this is usually addressed by stating that either party may terminate the agreement by providing a reasonable written notice, usually 30 – 90 days.

e Submit 2 copies of the Contract/Letter of Agreement for review to the Associate Dean for Finances.

f Once all changes have been made and the contract is approved for content, the Associate Dean for Finances will give the 2 copies to the Associate Dean for Faculty and Clinical Affairs for signature. This may be done concurrently as Research Departmental approval is sought.

XIII Institutional Review Board (IRB) Approval or WMed Privacy Board Approval

a Following WMed Research Committee final approval your research *may not* begin until an Institutional Review Board or the WMed Privacy Board has approved your protocol.

b Submit to WMed Research Department a copy of your IRB approval when received.

XIV Signatures and Contact Information for all Investigators

Signatures and contact information must be provided on the submission form for all investigators of the study to assure compliance with regulatory policy.

Original Effective Date: 2/01/2002
Revision Date: 10/06/06

Western Michigan University School of Medicine Clinical Research Committee
Clinical Research Protocol Reviewer's Approval
Protocol Score Sheet

Protocol Title:
Principle Investigator:

	Yes	No	N/A
REVIEW OF LITERATURE			
Has a review of the literature been performed? Comments:			
HYPOTHESIS/SPECIFIC AIMS			
Is the hypothesis clearly stated in the protocol? Comments:			
METHODOLOGY/STUDY DESIGN			
Is the methodology and study design appropriate to validate the hypothesis/aims? Comments:			
SUBJECT ENROLLMENT			
Are the inclusion/exclusion criteria and subject population appropriate? Comments:			
Is the randomization process clearly described? Comments:			
Does the study satisfactorily address the inclusion of minorities/women/children? Comments:			
PATIENT SAFETY			
Is the risk/benefit ratio appropriate for this study? Comments:			
STATISTICAL ANALYSIS			
Is the power/sample size defined? Comments:			
DATA COLLECTION			
Does the protocol appropriately describe how the data will be stored and kept confidential? Comments:			

COMMENTS

Summarize the scientific concerns that must be addressed by the investigator to achieve Research Committee approval:

RECOMMENDATION

	Approved as presented. Procedures are consistent with sound scientific design, no revisions, restrictions or contingencies required by the Committee
	Modification(s) required. Protocol requires modifications that, when submitted, may be approved after an expedited review by the Chair and/or designated Research Committee members.

Reviewer: ______________________ Date: ______________

Western Michigan University School of Medicine
Clinical Research Committee
Research Proposal Final Approval

Title of Protocol:
Name of Investigators:

	Signature	**Date**
Research Committee protocol review for scientific merit satisfactory		
Documentation of completion of: Human Participant Protection Education Privacy Rule (HIPPA) for Research Financial Conflict of Interest Statement		
Human Resources Review		
Accounting Review		
Information Technology Review		
Final Institution Dean Designee Approval		

In: Principles of Research
Editor: Luis H. Toledo-Pereyra
ISBN: 978-1-62417-968-6

Appendix III

World Health Organization Recommended Format for a Research Protocol[1,*]

Luis H. Toledo-Pereyra
Western Michigan University School of Medicine,
Michigan State University College of Human Medicine,
Michigan State University College of Osteopathic Medicine,
Kalamazoo, MI, US

Part 1

Project summary -Like the abstract of a research paper, the project summary, should be no more than 300 words and at the most a page long (font size 12, single spacing). Provided preferably on a separate page, it should summarize all the central elements of the protocol, for example the rationale, objectives, methods, populations, time frame, and expected outcomes. It should stand on its own, and not refer the reader to points in the project description.

General information

- Protocol title, protocol identifying number (if any), and date.

---

[1] Obtained from the internet site of the "World Health Organization Recommended Format for a Research Protocol". Permission for publication granted on June 19, 2013 by Dolores Campanario, World Health Organization, Geneva, Switzerland.

- Name and address of the sponsor/funder.
- Name and title of the investigator(s) who is(are) responsible for conducting the research, and the address and telephone number(s) of the research site(s), including responsibilities of each.
- Name(s) and address(s) of the clinical laboratory(s) and other medical and/or technical department(s) and/or institutions involved in the research

Rationale & background information - The Rationale specifies the reasons for conducting the research in light of current knowledge. It should include a well documented statement of the need/problem that is the basis of the project, the cause of this problem and its possible solutions. It is the equivalent to the introduction in a research paper and it puts the proposal in context. It should answer the question of why and what: why the research needs to be done and what will be its relevance. The magnitude, frequency, affected geographical areas, ethnic and gender considerations, etc of the problem should be followed by a brief description of the most relevant studies published on the subject.

References (of literature cited in preceding sections) - References can also be listed at the end of Part 1.

Study goals and objectives - Goals are broad statements of what the proposal hopes to accomplish. They create a setting for the proposal. Specific objectives are statements of the research question(s). Objectives should be simple (not complex), specific (not vague), and stated in advance (not after the research is done). After statement of the primary objective, secondary objectives may be mentioned.

Study Design - The scientific integrity of the study and the credibility of the study data depend substantially on the study design and methodology. The design of the study should include information on the type of study, the research population or the sampling frame, and who can take part (e.g. inclusion and exclusion criteria, withdrawal criteria etc.), and the expected duration of the study

(The same study can be described in several ways, and as complete a description of the study as possible should be provided. For example, a study may be described as being a basic science research, epidemiologic or social science research, it may also be described as observational or interventional; if observational, it may be either descriptive or analytic, if analytic it could either be cross-sectional or longitudinal etc. If experimental, it may be described as a controlled or a non controlled study.

Methodology - The methodology section is the most important part of the protocol. It should include detailed information on the interventions to be made, procedures to be used, measurements to be taken, observations to be made, laboratory investigations to be done etc. If multiple sites are engaged in a specified protocol, methodology should be standardized and clearly defined.Interventions should be described in detail, including a description of the drug/device/vaccine that is being tested. Interventions could also be in the realm of social sciences for example providing training or information to groups of individuals.

Procedures could be biomedical (collection of blood or sputum samples to develop a diagnostic test), or in the realm of social sciences (doing a questionnaire survey, carrying out a focus group discussion as part of formative research, observation of the participant's environment, etc.).

Standardized and/or documented procedures/techniques should be described and bibliographic references, if not provided earlier should be provided. Instruments which are to be used to collect information (questionnaires, FGD guides, observation recording form, case report forms etc.) must also be provided.

In the case of a randomized controlled trial additional information on the process of randomization and blinding, description of stopping rules for individuals, for part of the study or entire study, the procedures and conditions for breaking the codes etc. should also be described.

A graphic outline of the study design and procedures using a flow diagram must be provided. This should include the timing of assessments.

Safety Considerations - The safety of research participants is foremost. Safety aspects of the research should always be kept in mind and information provided in the protocol on how the safety of research participants will be ensured. This can include procedures for recording and reporting adverse events and their follow-up, for example. It is useful to remember that even administering a research questionnaire can have adverse effects on individuals.

Follow-Up - The research protocol must give a clear indication of what follow up will be provided to the research participants and for how long. This may include a follow u, especially for adverse events, even after data collection for the research study is completed.

Data Management and Statistical Analysis - The protocol should provide information on how the data will be managed, including data handling and coding for computer analysis, monitoring and verification. The statistical methods proposed to be used for the analysis of data should be clearly outlined, including reasons for the sample size selected, power of the study, level of significance to be used, procedures for accounting for any missing or spurious data etc. For projects involving qualitative approaches, specify in sufficient detail how the data will be analyzed.

Quality Assurance - The protocol should describe the quality control and quality assurance system for the conduct of the study, including GCP, follow up by clinical monitors, DSMB, data management etc.

Expected Outcomes of the Study - The protocol should indicate how the study will contribute to advancement of knowledge, how the results will be utilized, not only in publications but also how they will likely affect health care, health systems, or health policies.

Dissemination of Results and Publication Policy - The protocol should specify not only dissemination of results in the scientific media, but also to the community and/ or the participants, and consider dissemination to the policy makers where relevant. Publication policy should be clearly discussed- for example who will take the lead in publication and who will be acknowledged in publications, etc.

Duration of the Project - The protocol should specify the time that each phase of the project is likely to take, along with a detailed month by month timeline for each activity to be undertaken.

Problems Anticipated - This section should discuss the difficulties that the investigators anticipate in successfully completing their projects within the time frame stipulated and the funding requested. It should also offer possible solutions to deal with these difficulties.

Project Management - This section should describe the role and responsibility of each member of the team

Ethics - The protocol should have a description of ethical considerations relating to the study. This should not be limited to providing information on how or from whom the ethics approval will be taken, but this section should document the issues that are likely to raise ethical concerns. It should also describe how the investigator(s) plan to obtain informed consent from the research participants (the informed consent process).

Informed Consent Forms - The approved version of the protocol must have copies of informed consent forms (ICF), both in English and the local language in which they are going to be administered. However translations may be carried out after the English language ICF(s) have been approved by the ERC. If the research involves more than one group of individuals, for example healthcare users and healthcare providers, a separate specifically tailored informed consent form must be included for each group. This ensures that each group of participants will get the information they need to make an informed decision. For the same reason, each new intervention also requires a separate informed consent form. For guidance on how to write an informed consent form, click here

Part 2

Budget - The budget section should contain a detailed item-wise breakdown of the funds requested for, along with a justification for each item.

Other support for the Project - This section should provide information about the funding received or anticipated for this project from other funding organizations.

Collaboration with other scientists or research institutions - Links to other projects

Curriculum Vitae of investigators - The CV of the Principal investigator and each co-investigators should be provided. In general each CV should not be more than one page, unless a complete CV is specifically requested for.

Other research activities of the investigators - The Principal investigator should list all current research projects that he/she is involved in, the source of funding of those projects, the duration of those projects and the percentage of time spent on each.

Financing and Insurance - Financing and insurance if not addressed in a separate agreement, and where relevant should be described.

In: Principles of Research
Editor: Luis H. Toledo-Pereyra
ISBN: 978-1-62417-968-6

Appendix IV

Clinical Trials Research[1]

Luis H. Toledo-Pereyra
Western Michigan University School of Medicine,
Michigan State University College of Human Medicine,
Michigan State University College of Osteopathic Medicine,
Kalamazoo, MI, US

The clinical trial is an important research design used to assess the safety and efficacy of new drugs, devices, treatments, or preventive measures in humans by comparing two or more interventions or regimens. Clinical trials are frequently "multicentered," that is, a number of research institutions may cooperate in a common study **protocol**.

Clinical trials can be used to evaluate most treatments or preventive measures for almost any condition or disease. Clinical trials (sometimes called "randomized clinical trials," or RCTs) are controlled (one subject group receives the treatment under investigation while a control subject group receives either another treatment or no treatment), with participants being randomly assigned to either the subject or control group. They are also either single- or double-masked, so that either the investigator, the subjects or both do not know who is in the treatment or control group until the conclusion of the study.

---

[1] Obtained in its entirety from the internet site of the *Institutional Review Board Guidebook* (updated 1993), from the United States Department of Health and Human Services and currently considered public domain.

Randomized clinical trials present numerous ethical issues, some of which are discussed in other Sections of this Guidebook as well as in this Section.

A primary ethical concern is one of fairness: If the trial therapy is known to be superior to currently available alternative therapies (*i.e.*, prior research indicates that it is superior), it is unethical to assign subjects to the inferior treatment. Furthermore, it would not be ethical to perform a clinical trial comparing two treatments when there is a third therapy that is known to be superior to either or both, unless there is some reason why that therapy is not useful for the study population. Researchers must therefore honestly be able to state a null hypothesis (also called "theoretical equipoise": the assumption that subjects treated with therapy A - the trial therapy - will not differ in outcome from subjects treated with therapy B - the control therapy) before beginning a randomized clinical trial [Freedman (1987)]. According to a somewhat broader concept called "clinical equipoise," a randomized controlled design may be justified where there is a "current or likely dispute among expert members of the clinical community as to which of two or more therapies is superior in all relevant respects" [Levine, Dubler, and Levine (1991), p. 3, restating Freedman (1987)]. Furthermore, the trial must be designed such that its "successful completion will show which [of the therapies] is superior" [Freedman (1990), p. 5]. The "results of a successful clinical trial should be convincing enough to resolve the dispute among physicians" [Freedman (1987), p. 144]. The control treatment must be the best standard therapy currently available for the condition being treated [Freedman (1990); Levine (1986), (1985)].

Placebos. Placebos may be used in clinical trials where there is no known or available (*i.e*, FDA-approved) alternative therapy that can be tolerated by subjects. IRBs should scrutinize studies that propose to use placebos to ensure that subjects are not deceived into believing that they have received an active agent.

Where the disease is lethal or seriously debilitating, however (as in the case of HIV), the use of a placebo control in place of an active control may be, and indeed has been, questioned. The onslaught of HIV has led to considerable discussion of clinical trial design and the need to maximize benefits in every arm of the trial. [*See, e.g.*, Levine, Dubler, and Levine (1991) and Freedman (1990).] A design involving a placebo control should not be used where there is a standard treatment that has been shown to be superior to placebo by convincing evidence [Freedman (1990)]. It has been argued that placebo controls must be used, however, when the experimental treatment is of "dubious efficacy" or when there are known serious side effects [Freedman (1990); Levine (1985), 1986)]. The use of placebos in controlled clinical trials must be justified by a positive risk-benefit analysis, and subjects must be fully informed of the risks involved in assignment to the placebo group. There is a consensus that continued assignment of subjects to placebo is unethical once there is good evidence to support the efficacy of the trial therapy. Clinical trials should be stopped or their protocols modified when there is sufficient evidence of either a beneficial therapeutic effect or unacceptable side effects. Monitoring for such information during the course of the trial is discussed in Guidebook Chapter 3, Section E, "Monitoring and Observation."

Some drug trials involve a period during which all subjects receive only a placebo prior to the initiation of the study. This period is called a "placebo washout." The purposes of a washout period include: (1) terminating the effects of any drug the subject may have been taking before entering the clinical trial, so that the effects of the trial drug - and only the trial drug - may be observed; (2) learning whether subjects cooperate with instructions to take drugs ("compliance"); and (3) learning which subjects are "placebo responders," in that they experience a high degree of placebo effect. In some protocols, the investigators plan to exclude those subjects they find either poorly compliant or highly responsive to the placebo. The risks entailed in withdrawing subjects from therapy during a placebo washout period should be carefully evaluated by the IRB; great care must be taken to exclude subjects who are vulnerable to injury if they are withdrawn from effective therapy. In studies involving a placebo washout, subjects should be told that at some point during the study all subjects will receive placebo treatment; investigators but not subjects will know when subjects are receiving placebos for washout purposes, so that during the washout, the study is single-masked.

Informed consent. Informed consent is of particular importance in randomized clinical trials as in all **prospective studies**. The IRB should assure that initial, and, where necessary, continuing consent is obtained from the subjects at critical intervals (*e.g*., at points where the study protocol is materially altered, new procedures are introduced, new information - about risks or benefits, for instance - becomes available, or toxicity becomes manifest). In such instances, blanket consent at the beginning of the study does not suffice. Because subjects may forget crucial aspects of the trial, it may also be advisable periodically to ascertain continuing consent in long-term studies.

Despite the fact that subjects may be kept unaware of their treatment assignments in "masked" studies and research involving placebos, the information provided to prospective subjects should clearly communicate the nature of the study design, method of treatment assignment (including the probability of assignment to the various groups), possible interventions, and the implications of the possible interventions. Ethical considerations demand that subjects be informed when their assignment will be **random**, and that one of the possible consequences of participation is that the group to which they are assigned will turn out to have received the less effective intervention.

Subjects must be fully informed of the likelihood of receiving the experimental treatment. For example, if there are two subject groups, experimental and control, and the assignment of subjects to groups is random, subjects must be informed that they have a 50 percent chance of receiving the experimental therapy and a 50 percent chance of receiving the alternative treatment. **If the alternative "treatment" is placebo, subjects must be so informed.** Informing subjects that the study involves the use of placebos and the probability of their being assigned to the placebo group eliminates the ethically objectionable element of deception from the study. Further, subjects should be told who will know whether they are receiving the placebo or the active agent. In a double-masked trial, for example, subjects should be told that neither they nor the investigator will know whether they are receiving the placebo or the experimental therapy.

Since assignment to one or another of the interventions should take place after informed consent has been given, the subject must be made aware of all the possible alternative interventions and what is known about the efficacy and safety of each. Prospective subjects should also be told whether participation in the study precludes participation in other programs or therapeutic regimens that may be beneficial to them and the extent to which this restriction presents a risk.

A more fundamental consent question centers on communicating the uncertainties and risks involved in clinical trials to prospective subjects. Particularly in Phase 1 trials, where the safety of therapies in humans is first being tested, IRBs must assure themselves that those risks and uncertainties will be clearly communicated to prospective subjects, and that the process of communication with subjects will continue throughout the study.

A related issue is the selection of subjects. Subjects who are particularly vulnerable, such as persons who are desperately ill, are, perhaps, more likely than others to be willing to accept great risks in the hope that they will benefit from an experimental treatment. IRBs need to ensure that their welfare is protected by requiring full and open disclosure of risks and benefits, while at the same time avoiding paternalism. Vulnerable subjects should not be precluded from studies solely on the basis of their vulnerability. To do so would preclude them from the opportunity to benefit from the availability of investigational therapies through research studies. [*See* also Guidebook Chapter 3, Section A, "Risk/Benefit Analysis," Chapter 3, Section C, "Selection of Subjects," Chapter 5, "Biomedical and Behavioral Research," and Chapter 6, "Special Classes of Subjects."]

IDENTIFICATION AND RECRUITMENT OF SUBJECTS

This Section deals specifically with practical aspects of how investigators go about identifying and recruiting individual subjects, and IRB considerations related to these activities. These considerations are especially important in **epidemiologic** research.

See also Guidebook Chapter 3, Section C, "Selection of Subjects," and Chapter 3, Section G, "Incentives for Participation." "Selection of Subjects" deals with the question of equitable selection of subjects in terms of defining the appropriate group of subjects for a research project. "Incentives for Participation" deals in greater depth than the present Section with incentives offered to encourage participation and the ethical concerns of coercion and undue influence.

IRB CONSIDERATIONS

Using Records to Identify Subjects. IRBs are responsible for ensuring the equitable selection of research subjects [Federal Policy §___.111(a)(3)]. In fulfilling this responsibility, IRBs should review the methods that investigators use to recruit subjects.

Subjects with specific diseases or conditions are often identified as potential subjects through some type of record (*e.g.*, registries for cancer cases, surgical or X-ray log books, employment or school records). **Controls** may come from the same population as the subjects (which is always the case in a randomized clinical trial), be persons with unrelated conditions or be volunteers from the general population. Potential subjects may be identified through records maintained at hospitals or physicians' private offices. If potential subjects are identified through medical records, log books, physicians' records, or other records that are not public documents, the IRB should make certain that the following conditions have been met: (1) the investigator is allowed access to such records by the institution or the physician; and (2) responsibility for **confidentiality** and protection of **privacy** is clearly accepted by the investigator.

Sometimes, as in epidemiologic research, it is necessary for an investigator to review thousands of medical records to identify a very small number of subjects who are suitable for a study. At present, there is no agreement among commentators as to whether the investigator needs **consent** from all patients whose records will be searched, or only from the few who are selected for the study. An alternative in some circumstances may be the use of a "data broker," that is, an intermediary who already has access to the data. The broker can review records to identify appropriate subjects, whose consent to participate in the study can then be sought. With automated record keeping systems, it may be easier to identify appropriate subjects without reviewing all the records. Where the records are not computerized, however, IRBs will have to decide under what conditions a scientist may scan thousands of medical or other private records while searching for a small number of appropriate subjects. One factor to consider would be the sensitivity of the information likely to be contained in the records. For example, did the patients have broken ankles or abortions? Were they treated for strep throat or venereal disease? Another factor to consider is the type of information the investigator wishes to obtain from those who are selected as suitable subjects for the study.

Some institutions notify patients at the time of admission or initial treatment that: (1) their records may be used for research purposes; and (2) precautions will be taken to ensure that if the records are used, the researchers will respect and protect the confidentiality of the records. Some institutions go further and provide an opportunity for patients to consent or refuse consent to such use of their records at the time of admission.

In the event that names are sought from physicians' private offices, the patient's physician should request permission from the patient to release his or her name.

For a hospital-based study, most IRBs require that a potential subject's physician give approval before the subject is contacted, particularly when there may be medical or emotional contraindications to participation. If the subject is in the hospital, someone on the hospital staff may inform the patient that he or she is going to be invited to participate in a study, or, more often, an interviewer may approach the subject directly after consultation with his or her physician.

If the subject has left the hospital, various options may be considered. (For each option, most IRBs require that the potential subject's physician give approval before the subject is contacted.) For instance, the investigator may send a letter describing the purpose of the study and requesting that the subject return a postcard indicating whether he or she would like to participate. The effectiveness of this method depends on how many of the postcards are returned.

A second option is to invite participation by letter, and for the subject to send back a postcard (or to telephone) only if he or she does not wish to participate. If no postcard is returned, the subject may then be contacted by an interviewer. This method is less preferable, as it requires that potential subjects take positive action to avoid being made part of a study rather than the other way around. Subjects may become unwitting participants if, for example, they never receive the letter, don't read English, or are simply confused by the instructions. This approach also raises **privacy** concerns for certain types of research (*e.g.*, research involving sexually transmitted diseases or psychiatric illness, or drug or alcohol abuse).

A third approach that is often used is for the patient's physician to send a letter informing the subject about the study and inviting the patient to participate. This method may work well if the study is being undertaken by a relatively small number of physicians who are willing to cooperate with the investigator. Response rates are likely to be high, since the subject often considers it significant that the letter has come from his or her own physician. IRBs should consider whether use of this method will subject potential participants to coercion or undue influence. Finally, the investigator can send a letter to the potential subject explaining the purpose of the study, and then an interviewer can call to invite the potential subject to participate. By permitting interchange between the subject and interviewer, this method allows the subject to make an informed decision about participation. Although there is the risk of coercion by the interviewer, in general this method helps the subject better understand what the purposes of the research are, why his or her participation is important, what procedures are used to protect confidentiality, and what would be asked of him or her as a participant. This approach usually secures the highest response rate; however, people may be offended, especially in research on sensitive topics, by the investigator's having direct access to their name, address, and phone number. IRBs should be sensitive to this concern.

Advertising for Subjects. One method of recruiting subjects is through advertisements (*e.g.*, posted notices and newspaper or magazine ads). Advertising for research subjects is not, in and of itself, an objectionable practice. When advertising is to be used, however, the FDA requests that IRBs review the information contained in the advertisement, as well as the mode of its communication, to determine whether the procedure for recruiting subjects affords adequate protection. IRB review is necessary to ensure that the information is not misleading to subjects, especially when a study will involve persons with acute or severe physical or mental illness, or persons who are economically or educationally disadvantaged.

The FDA believes that any advertisement to recruit subjects should be limited to: (1) the name and address of the clinical investigator; (2) the purpose of the research, and, in summary form, the eligibility criteria that will be used to admit subjects into the study; (3) a straightforward and truthful description of the incentives to the subject for participation in the study (*e.g.*, payments or free treatment); and (4) the location of the research and the person to contact for further information [*FDA IRB Information Sheet*: "Advertising For Study Subjects" (1989)].

If a study involves investigational drugs or devices, no claims should be made, either explicitly or implicitly, that the drug or device is safe or effective for the purposes under investigation, or that the drug or device is in any way equivalent or superior to any other drug or device. Such representation would not only be misleading to subjects, but would also violate FDA regulations concerning the promotion of investigational drugs [21 CFR 312.7(a)] and investigational devices [21 CFR 812.7(d)].

Paying Subjects to Participate. Another method of recruiting research subjects is to pay them for their participation. It is not uncommon for subjects to be paid for their participation in research, especially in the early phases of investigational drug or device development. In such cases, the IRB should review both the amount of payment and the proposed method of disbursement to assure that neither entails problems of coercion or undue influence. Such problems might occur, for example, if the entire payment were to be contingent upon completion of the study or if the payment were unusually large. Payments should reflect the degree of risk, inconvenience, or discomfort associated with participation. *See* Guidebook Chapter 3, Section G, "Incentives for Participation."

ASSIGNMENT OF SUBJECTS TO EXPERIMENTAL AND CONTROL GROUPS

Introduction

The choice of study design depends largely upon the nature and goals of the research. Good methodology requires that studies be designed to minimize bias both in assignment to treatment groups (*e.g.*, by randomizing) and in assessment of outcome. Bias may enter into a study in several ways. The investigator may have strong beliefs or hopes regarding the success of a particular intervention or the truth of a particular hypothesis; these expectations may unconsciously influence his or her evaluation of the outcome of the research. To avoid this possibility, it is now accepted and preferred practice to conduct controlled investigations by dividing subjects into at least two groups: those who receive the experimental intervention (the experimental or treatment group) and those who do not (the control group).

IRB Considerations

Random Assignment. To minimize the possibility that investigators may consciously or unconsciously select one sort of subject (*e.g.*, the most intelligent or the least sick) for the experimental group, it has become accepted and preferred practice to devise methods of randomly assigning subjects to experimental and control groups, unless there are important scientific or ethical reasons to do otherwise. The justifying pre-condition for ethical use of randomization is that a **null hypothesis** (*i.e.*, the stated experimental hypothesis that the experimental and control conditions have equally beneficial effects) can be reasonably entertained.

Sometimes experimental subjects and control subjects are assigned to groups upon admission to the study and remain in those groups for the duration of the study. This design is called "parallel control." On the other hand, it is sometimes advisable to let each subject be his or her own control by having the subject be on both regimens - first the experimental treatment and then the control, or vice versa. This "**cross-over design**" can be useful because it reduces variability (since every subject receives both the experimental intervention and the control treatment) and it requires fewer subjects.

Several conditions are required for the cross-over design to be appropriate. First, the condition or disease must be stable, and, if relieved, not permanently cured by either the intervention or control. Second, there must be no "carry-over" effect from the first to the second treatment assignment (*e.g.*, in a drug study, sufficient time must elapse between treatments to ensure that all traces of the first treatment have been eliminated). Unfortunately, it is often difficult to demonstrate that these conditions exist.

Regardless of the type of design, random assignment of subjects to treatment groups is generally the preferred method in most controlled studies. Random assignment is preferred because other techniques hold the opportunity for bias in the selection of subjects for particular treatments. Assigning every other consenting subject to a given treatment or assigning subjects to a treatment group based on the day of hospital admission are not truly random methods of assignment.

In situations where the course of the disease (under currently available standard treatment) is so clear or well-known that randomization is not ethically possible (*see* Guidebook Chapter 4, Section H, "Clinical Trials"), a *historical control* design may be an alternative design choice. In historically controlled studies, the condition of subjects is compared with their own past condition on a prior regimen or treatment. For example, if a disease is known to be fatal in 80 percent of the cases and no conventional therapy exists, an experimental treatment with a good chance of success (*e.g.*, based on the results of animal studies) might be offered to all eligible subjects identified by the investigators. It may not be ethically acceptable to ask subjects to accept the possibility of assignment to a control (untreated) group if the null hypothesis cannot reasonably be entertained.

In some circumstances, however, the use of historical controls can yield erroneous conclusions. Because changing standards of hygiene, lifestyle patterns, and medical care can markedly alter the course of a disease, the use of historical controls to demonstrate the effectiveness of a new treatment could be misleading. Small effects are particularly difficult to detect with such designs.

Placebos. To minimize the possibility that the investigators' beliefs or hopes regarding the outcome of the research will bias their evaluation of the subjects' responses, investigators may be kept unaware of the identity of subjects who are assigned to each treatment group. Similarly, the subjects' hopes for a "cure" for a disease or their fears of side effects may cause them to experience improvement or adverse effects unrelated to the experimental treatment. Furthermore, it is generally agreed that a substantial number of patients will experience improvement in their symptoms regardless of treatment. To reduce the possibility that subjects' responses will result from their expectations rather than the interventions under study, it has become accepted and preferred practice to have subjects be unaware whether the "treatment" they are given is the experimental intervention. In **clinical trials**, control subjects may be given either a conventional treatment, or, if none is available or appropriate, a **placebo** - an inert substance prepared to resemble an experimental drug in size, shape, color, taste, etc. The use of placebos is generally unacceptable if there is an effective therapy that the subjects could be receiving for relief of severe symptoms or amelioration of a serious condition. [*See* also Guidebook Chapter 3, Section B, "Informed Consent," and Chapter 4, Section H, "Clinical Trials."]

Some drug trials involve a period during which all subjects receive only a placebo prior to the initiation of the study. This period is called a "placebo washout." The purposes of a washout period include: (1) terminating the effects of any drug the subject may have been taking before entering the clinical trial, so that the effects of the trial drug - and only the trial drug - may be observed; (2) learning whether subjects cooperate with instructions to take drugs ("compliance"); and (3) learning which subjects are "placebo responders," in that they experience a high degree of placebo effect. In some protocols, the investigators plan to exclude those subjects they find either poorly compliant or highly responsive to the placebo. The risks entailed in withdrawing subjects from therapy during a placebo washout period should be carefully evaluated by the IRB; great care must be taken to exclude subjects who are vulnerable to injury if they are withdrawn from effective therapy. In studies involving a placebo washout, subjects should be told that at some point during the study all subjects will receive placebo treatment; investigators but not subjects will know when subjects are receiving placebos for washout purposes, so that during the washout, the study is single-masked.

When both the investigator and the subjects are unaware of the treatment assignments, the design is called "**double-masked**;" when one or the other (but not both) know, it is called "**single-masked**." Whenever the investigator remains unaware of the treatment that subjects are receiving, it is important that someone be able to find out, in case it becomes necessary to protect the health and well-being of a subject (*i.e.*, in case of serious adverse effect or deterioration of a patient's condition). Therefore, investigators usually arrange for an independent person to have access to a code indicating the identity of subjects assigned to each treatment. This independent person is given the authority to break the code for individual subjects in case of emergency. This arrangement permits treatment to be provided, as necessary, to a particular subject without breaking the "masked" aspect of the experimental design. The protocol should describe how these arrangements will be made. [*See* also Guidebook Chapter 4, Section H, "Clinical Trials."]

POINTS TO CONSIDER

1. Does the study involve reviews of records, observation, surveys, or interviews? If so, does it qualify for exemption or expedited review under the federal regulations and institutional policy?
2. Is the scientific design adequate to answer the questions posed? Is the sample size (number of subjects) adequate? Is the method proposed for selecting and assigning subjects to treatment groups unbiased?
3. Does the investigator serve a dual role that may pose a conflict of interest?
4. Is any of the information to be collected sensitive (*e.g.*, related to sexual practices, substance abuse, or illegal behavior)?
5. Are there adequate plans to protect participants from the risks of breach of confidentiality and invasion of privacy?
6. Are there plans for approaching subjects in a way that will respect their privacy and their right to refuse? If the protocol involves an epidemiologic study, will subjects or their relatives be protected from learning inappropriate information?
7. Does the recruitment process protect subjects from being coerced or unduly influenced to participate? Are any payments to subjects reasonable in relation to the risks, discomfort, or inconvenience to which subjects will be exposed?
8. Are there adequate plans to exclude subjects who are vulnerable to injury during the period of withdrawal of active and effective therapy, if that is part of the research design?
9. Have the rights and interests of vulnerable subjects (*e.g.*, desperately ill persons) been adequately considered?
10. Are all appropriate elements of informed consent clearly provided for [Federal Policy §____.116], including:
    a. Do the consent documents describe the study design (including plans for randomization, use of placebos, and the probability that the subject will receive a given treatment) and conditions for breaking the code (if the study is masked)?

b. Do the consent documents describe the risks and benefits of each of the proposed interventions and of alternative courses or actions available to the participants?
c. Do the consent documents clearly describe the extent to which participation in the study precludes other therapeutic interventions?
d. Are provisions made for supplying new information to subjects during the course of the study and for obtaining continuing consent, where appropriate?
e. Must investigators obtain consent before reviewing records?

11. Will the consent process take place under conditions most likely to provide potential subjects an opportunity to make a decision about participation without undue pressure?
12. If the study is a clinical trial, how will the trial be monitored? What will be done with preliminary data? Should an independent data and safety monitoring board be established? How will decisions about stopping the trial be made? By whom? On what basis?
13. At what interval should the IRB perform continuing review of this project?

SUGGESTIONS FOR FURTHER READING

Ackerman, Terrance F. "An Ethical Framework for the Practice of Paying Research Subjects." *IRB* 11 (No. 4, July/August 1989): 1-4.

Adelson, Julie Gross; Chiazze, Leonard, Jr.; Weintraub, Alan; and Walters, LeRoy. "The Use of Medical Records for Research at Georgetown University." *IRB* 3 (No. 3, March 1981): 1-3.

American Psychological Association. *Ethical Principles in the Conduct of Research with Human Participants*. Washington, D.C.: American Psychological Association, 1982.

Appelbaum, Paul S. et al. "Researchers' Access to Patient Records: An Analysis of the Ethical Problems." *Clinical Research* 32 (No. 4, October 1984): 399-403.

Arpaillange, P., and Dion, S. "The Ethical Approach to Randomization in Oncology." *Drugs Under Experimental and Clinical Research* 12 (No. 1/2/3, 1986): 99-103.

Arvino, Andrew, and Lo, Bernard. "To Tell or Not to Tell: The Ethical Dilemmas of HIV Test Notification in Epidemiologic Research." *American Journal of Public Health* 79 (No. 11, 1989): 1544-48.

Australia. *National Medical Council.* Report on Ethics in Epidemiological Research. Canberra: Australian Government Publishing Service, 1985.

Barlow, David H.; Hayes, Steven C.; and Nelson, Rosemary O. "Issues, Ethics, and Examples in the Use of Time-Series Methodology in Practice." *In The Scientist Practitioner: Research and Accountability in Clinical and Educational Settings*, edited by David H. Barlow, Steven C. Hayes, and Rosemary O. Nelson, pp. 273-289. New York: Pergamon Press, 1984.

Baumrind, Diana. "Research Using Intentional Deception: Ethical Issues Revisited." *American Psychologist* 40 (No. 2, February 1985): 165-74.

Bayer, Ronald; Levine, Carol; and Murray, Thomas H. "Guidelines for Confidentiality in Research on AIDS." *IRB* 6 (No. 6, November/December 1984): 1-9.

Beauchamp, Tom L. "Ethical Theory and Epidemiology." *Journal of Clinical Epidemiology* 44 (Supp. I, 1991): 5s-8s.

Beauchamp, Tom L. et al. "Appendix: Ethical Guidelines for Epidemiologists." *Journal of Clinical Epidemiology* 44 (Supp. I, 1991): 151s-169s.

Beauchamp, Tom L.; Faden, Ruth R.; Wallace, R. Jay, Jr.; and Walters, LeRoy, eds. *Ethical Issues in Social Science Research.* Baltimore, MD: Johns Hopkins University Press, 1982.

Boring, E. G. *A History of Experimental Psychology*. New York: Appleton-Century-Crafts, 1950.

Boruch, Robert F. "Methods for Resolving Privacy Problems in Social Research." *In Ethical Issues in Social Science Research*, edited by Tom L. Beauchamp, Ruth R. Faden, R. Jay Wallace, Jr., and LeRoy Walters, pp. 292-314. Baltimore, MD: Johns Hopkins University Press, 1982.

Brazzell, Romulus K., and Colburn, Wayne A. "Controversy I: Patients or Healthy Volunteers for Pharmacokinetic Studies?" *Journal of Clinical Pharmacology* 26 (No. 4, April 1986): 242-254.

Brett, A., and Grodin, M. "Ethical Aspects of Human Experimentation in Health Services Research." *Journal of the American Medical Association* 265 (No. 14, April 10, 1991): 1854-1857.

Buck, Beverly A. "Ethical Issues of Randomized Clinical Trials." *Radiologic Technology* 61 (No. 3, January/February 1990): 202-205.

Cann, Cristina I., and Rothman, Kenneth J. "IRBs and Epidemiologic Research: How Inappropriate Restrictions Hamper Studies." *IRB* 6 (No. 4, July/August 1984): 5-7.

Cann, Cristina I., and Rothman, Kenneth J. "Reply: Overcoming Hurdles to Epidemiologic Research." *IRB* 7 (No. 2, March/April 1985): 9. This article is a reply to Nathan Hershey, "IRB Jurisdiction and Limits on IRB Actions," *IRB* 7 (No. 2, March/April 1985): 7-9.

Caplan, Arthur L. "Is There an Obligation to Participate in Biomedical Research?" *In The Use of Human Beings in Research*, edited by Stuart F. Spicker, Ilai Alan, Andre de Vries, and H. Tristam Engelhardt, Jr., pp. 229-248. Boston: Kluwer Academic, 1988.

Capron, A.M. "Protection of Research Subjects: Do Special Rules Apply in Epidemiology?" *Journal of Clinical Epidemiology* 44 (Supp. I, 1991): 81s-89s. Reprinted in *Law, Medicine and Health Care* 19 (No. 3-4, Fall/Winter 1991): 184-190.

Chalmers, Thomas C. "Ethical Implications of Rejecting Patients for Clinical Trials." *Journal of the American Medical Association* 263 (No. 6, February 9, 1990): 865.

Chalmers, Thomas. "The Ethics of Randomization as a Decision-Making Technique and the Problem of Informed Consent." *In Contemporary Issues in Bioethics*, edited by Tom Beauchamp and LeRoy Walters, pp. 426-429. Belmont, CA: Wadsworth Publishing Co., 1978.

Cobb, L.A. et al. "An Evaluation of Internal Mammary Artery Ligation by a Double Blind Technique." *New England Journal of Medicine* 260 (No. 22, May 28, 1959): 1115-1118.

Conner, Ross F. "Random Assignments of Clients in Social Experimentation." *In The Ethics of Social Research: Surveys and Experiments*, edited by Joan E. Sieber, pp. 57-77. New York: Springer-Verlag, 1982.

Council for International Organizations of Medical Sciences (CIOMS). *International Guidelines for Ethical Review of Epidemiological Studies*. Geneva: Council for International Organizations of Medical Sciences, 1991. Reprinted in *Law, Medicine and Health Care* 19 (No. 3-4, Fall/Winter 1991): 247-58.

Cowan, Dale H. "Scientific Design, Ethics and Monitoring: IRB Review of Randomized Clinical Trials." *IRB* 2 (No. 9, November 1980): 1-4.

Culliton, B.J. "Human Experimentation: AIDS Trials Questioned." *Nature* 350 (No. 6316, March 28, 1991): 263.

Cowan, D.H. "IRB Review of Randomized Clinical Trials." *IRB* 2 (No. 9, November 1980): 1.

Drew, Clifford J., and Hardman, Michael L. "Ethical Issues in Conducting Research." *In Designing and Conducting Behavioral Research*, edited by Clifford J. Drew and Michael L. Hardman, pp. 29-48. New York: Pergamon Press, 1985.

Dubler, Nancy N., and Sidel, Victor W. "On Research on HIV Infection in Correctional Institutions." *Milbank Quarterly* 67 (No. 2, 1989): 171-207.

Durry, G., and Dion, S. "The Ethical Approach to Phase I Clinical Trials in Oncology." *Drugs Under Experimental and Clinical Research* 12 (Nos. 1/2/3, 1986): 21-22.

Ellenberg, Susan S. "Randomization Designs in Comparative Clinical Trials." *New England Journal of Medicine* 310 (No. 21, May 24, 1984): 1404-1408.

Engelhardt, H. Tristram. "Diagnosing Well and Treating Prudently: Randomized Clinical Trials and the Problem of Knowing Truly." *In The Use of Human Beings in Research*, edited by Stuart F. Spicker, Ilai Alan, Andre de Vries, and H. Tristam Engelhardt, Jr., pp. 123-141. Boston: Kluwer Academic, 1988.

Finkel, Marion J. "Should Informed Consent Include Information on How Research is Funded?" *IRB* 13 (No. 5, September/October 1991): 1-3.

Freedman, Benjamin. "Placebo-Controlled Trials and the Logic of Clinical Purpose." *IRB* 12 (No. 6, November/December 1990):1-6.

Freedman, Benjamin. "Equipoise and the Ethics of Clinical Research." *New England Journal of Medicine* 317 (No. 3, July 16, 1987): 141-145.

Freedman, Benjamin. "Scientific Value and Validity as Ethical Requirements for Research: A Proposed Explication." *IRB* 9 (No. 6, November/ December 1987): 7-10.

Fried, Charles. "Informed Consent and Medical Experimentation." *In Contemporary Issues in Bioethics*, edited by Tom Beauchamp and LeRoy Walters, pp. 436-441. Belmont, CA: Wadsworth Publishing Co., 1978.

Fried, Charles. *Medical Experimentation: Personal Integrity and Social Policy*. New York: American Elsevier Company, 1974.

Friedman, Gary D. *Primer of Epidemiology*, 2d ed. New York: McGraw-Hill, 1980.

Friedman, L.F.; Furberg, C.; and DeMets, D. *Fundamentals of Clinical Trials*. Boston: Wright-PSG, 1981.

Geller, Daniel M. "Alternatives to Deception: Why, What, and How?" *In The Ethics of Social Research: Surveys and Experiments*, edited by Joan E. Sieber, pp. 39-55. New York: Springer-Verlag, 1982.

Giammona, Mary, and Glantz, Stanton A. "Poor Statistical Design in Research on Humans: The Role of Committees in Human Research." *Clinical Research* 31 (No. 5, December 1983): 572-578.

Gifford, Fred. "The Conflict between Randomized Clinical Trials and the Therapeutic Obligation." *Journal of Medicine and Philosophy* 11 (No. 4, November, 1986): 347-366.

Glover, Jonathan. "Questions About Some Uses of Genetic Engineering." *In Contemporary Issues in Bioethics*, edited by Tom Beauchamp and LeRoy Walters, pp. 525-535. Belmont, CA: Wadsworth Publishing Co., 1978.

Goldberg, H.I., and McGough, H. "The Ethics of Ongoing Randomization Trials: Investigation Among Intimates." *Medical Care* 29 (7 Supp., July 1991): JS41-JS48.

Gordis, Leon, and Gold, Ellen. "Privacy, Confidentiality and the Use of Medical Records in Research." *Science* 207 (January 11, 1980):153-156.

Gordon, Robert S., Jr. "The Design and Conduct of Randomized Clinical Trials." *IRB* 7 (No. 1, January/February 1985): 1-3, 12.

Gostin, Larry. "Ethical Principles for the Conduct of Human Subject Research: Population-Based Research and Ethics." *Law, Medicine and Health Care* 19 (No. 3-4, Fall/Winter 1991): 191-201.

Great Britain. Medical Research Council. "Responsibility in the Use of Personal Medical Information for Research: Principles and Guide to Practice." *British Medical Journal* 290 (April 13, 1985): 1120-1124.

Guyatt, Gordon Guyatt et al. "Determining Optimal Therapy - Randomized Trials in Individual Patients." *New England Journal of Medicine* 314 (No. 14, April 3, 1986): 889-892.

Hartley, Shirley Foster. "Sampling Strategies and the Threat to Privacy." *In The Ethics of Social Research: Surveys and Experiments*, edited by Joan E. Sieber, pp. 167-189. New York: Springer-Verlag, 1982.

Hermeren, Goran. "Ethical Problems in Register Based Medical Research." *Theoretical Medicine* 9 (No. 2, June 1988): 105-116.

Hershey, Nathan. "IRB Jurisdiction and Limits on IRB Actions." *IRB* 7 (No. 2, March/April 1985): 7-9. See also Christina I. Cann and Kenneth J. Rothman, "Reply: Overcoming Hurdles to Epidemiologic Research," *IRB* 7 (No. 2, March/April 1985): 9.

Hill, Austin Bradford. "Medical Ethics and Controlled Trials." *British Medical Journal* (No. 5337, April 20, 1963): 1043-1049. Reprinted in *Ethics in Medicine*, edited by Stanley J. Reiser, Arthur J. Dyck, and William J. Curran. Cambridge, MA: MIT Press, 1977.

Johnson, Nicholas; Lilford, Richard J.; and Brazier, Wayne. "At What Level of Collective Equipoise Does a Clinical Trial Become Ethical?" *Journal of Medical Ethics* 17 (No. 1, March 1991): 30-34.

Jonsen, Albert. "Randomized Clinical Trials." *Triangle* 19 (1980): 89.

Kadane, Joseph B. "Progress Toward a More Ethical Method for Clinical Trials." *Journal of Medicine and Philosophy* 11 (No. 4, November 1986): 385-404.

Kassirer, J.P. "Clinical Trials and Meta-Analysis C What Do They Do for Us?" *New England Journal of Medicine* 327 (No. 4, July 23, 1992): 273-274.

Kelsey, J.L. "Privacy and Confidentiality in Epidemiological Research Involving Patients." *IRB* 3 (No. 2, February 1981): 1-4.

Keppel, Geoffrey. *Design and Analysis: A Researcher's Handbook*. Englewood Cliffs, NJ: Prentice Hall, 1982.

Klerman, Gerald L. "Scientific and Ethical Considerations in the Use of Placebo Controls in Clinical Trials in Psychopharmacology." *Psychopharmacology Bulletin* 22 (No. 1, 1986): 25-29.

Kravitz, Richard. "Serving Several Masters: Conflicting Responsibilities in Health Services Research." *Journal of General Internal Medicine* 5 (No. 2, March/April 1990): 170-174.

Kopelman, Loretta. "Consent and Randomized Clinical Trials: Are There Moral or Design Problems?" *Journal of Medicine and Philosophy* 11 (No. 4, November 1986): 317-345.

L'Abbe, K.A.; Detsky, A.S.; and O'Rourke, K. "Meta-Analysis in Clinical Research." *Annals of Internal Medicine* 107 (No. 2, August 1987): 224-233.

Lackey, Douglas P. "A Single Subject in Multiple Protocols: Is the Risk Equitable?" *IRB* 8 (No. 1, January/February 1986): 8-10.

Last, John M. "Epidemiology and Ethics." *Law, Medicine and Health Care* 19 (No. 3-4, Fall/Winter 1991): 166-174.

Lau, J., et al. "Cumulative Meta-Analysis of Therapeutic Trials for Myocardial Infarction." *New England Journal of Medicine* 327 (No. 4, July 23, 1992): 248-254.

Levine, Robert J., and Lebacqz, Karen. "Some Ethical Considerations in Clinical Trials." *Clinical Pharmacology and Therapeutics* 25 (No. 5, Pt. 2, May 1979): 728-741. Remarks and commentary following on pp. 742-749.

Levine, Robert J. "The Use of Placebos in Randomized Clinical Trials." *IRB* 7 (No. 2, March/April 1985): 1-4. Comment by Arthur Schafer, p. 4.

Levine, Robert J. *Ethics and Regulation of Clinical Research.* 2d ed. Baltimore: Urban and Schwarzenberg, 1986. See Chapter 8, "Randomized Clinical Trials."

Levine, Robert J. "Uncertainty in Clinical Research." *Law, Medicine and Health Care* 16 (Nos. 3-4, Fall/Winter 1988): 174-182.

Lind, Stuart E. "Can Patients Be Asked to Pay for Experimental Treatment?" *Clinical Research* 32 (No. 4, October 1984): 393-398.

Lind, Stuart E. "Fee for Service Research." *New England Journal of Medicine* 314 (No. 5, January 30, 1986): 312-315.

Lind, Stuart E. "Dilemmas in Paying for Clinical Research: The View From the IRB." *IRB* 9 (No. 2, March/April 1987): 1-5.

Lind, Stuart E. "Finder's Fees for Research Subjects." *New England Journal of Medicine* 323 (No. 3, July 19, 1990): 192-195.

Lind, Stuart E. "The Institutional Review Board: An Evolving Ethics Committee." *The Journal of Clinical Ethics* 3 (No. 4, Winter 1992): 278-282. See also commentary in the same issue by Troyen A. Brennan ("Researcher as Witness," dealing with health services research, pp. 308-309).

Llewellyn-Thomas, H.A.; Thiel, E.C.; and Clark, R.M. "Patients Versus Surrogates: Whose Opinion Counts on Ethics Review Panels?" *Clinical Research* 37 (No. 3, September 1989): 501-505.

Macklin, Ruth. "The Paradoxical Case of Payment as Benefit to Subjects." *IRB* 11 (No. 6, November/December 1989): 1-3.

Mackillop, William J., and Johnston, Pauline A. "Ethical Problems in Clinical Research: The Need for Empirical Studies of the Clinical Trials Process." *Journal of Chronic Diseases* 39 (No. 3, 1986): 177-188.

McCarthy, Charles R., and Porter, Joan P. "Confidentiality: The Protection of Personal Data in Epidemiological and Clinical Research Trials." *Law, Medicine and Health Care* 19 (No. 3-4, Fall/Winter 1991): 238-241.

McCartney, James J. "Encephalitis and Ara-A." *Hastings Center Report* 8 (No. 6, 1978): 5-7.

McLarty, Jerry W. "How Many Subjects are Required for a Study?" *IRB* 9 (No. 5, September/October 1987): 1-3. Comment by Robert J. Levine, p. 3.

McMahon, F. Gilbert. "Reviewing Subject Recruitment: New Rules from Rockville." *IRB* 10 (No. 3, May/June 1988): 6-7.

Mahler, Mark D. "When to Obtain Informed Consent in Behavioral Research: A Study of Mother-Infant Bonding." *IRB* 8 (No. 3, May/June 1986): 7-11.

Makuch, Robert W., and Johnson, Mary F. "Dilemmas in the Use of Active Control Groups in Clinical Research." *IRB* 11 (No. 1, January/February 1989): 1-5.

Markman, Maurie. "The Ethical Dilemma of Phase I Clinical Trials." *CA - A Cancer Journal for Clinicians* 36 (No. 6, November/December 1986): 367-369.

Marquis, Don. "An Argument that All Prerandomized Clinical Trials are Unethical." *Journal of Medicine and Philosophy* 11 (No. 4, November 1986): 367-383.

Marquis, Don et al. "When Research is Best Therapy." *Hastings Center Report* 18 (No. 2, April/May 1988): 24-26.

Meinert, Curtis L. *Clinical Trials: Design, Conduct, and Analysis*. New York and Oxford: Oxford University Press, 1986.

Melton, Gary B. "Ethical and Legal Issues in Research and Intervention." *Journal of Adolescent Health Care* 10 (Supp. 3, May 1989): 36S-44S.

Melton, Gary B. et al. "Community Consultation in Socially Sensitive Research: Lessons from Clinical Trials of Treatments for AIDS." *American Psychologist* 43 (No. 7, July 1988): 573-581.

Mitchell, Shiela C., and Steingrub, Jay. "The Changing Clinical Trials Scene: The Role of the IRB." *IRB* 10 (No. 4, July/August 1988): 1-5.

Morreim, E. Haavi. "Patient-Funded Research: Paying the Piper or Protecting the Patient?" *IRB* 13 (No. 3, May/June 1991): 1-6.

Myers, J. L. *Fundamentals of Experimental Design*. Boston: Allyn and Bacon, 1972.

Napier, Grace, ed. *Risk Assessment: Its Role in Health and Research*. Boston: Public Responsibility in Medicine and Research, 1981.

Newcomb, Polly A. and Rost, Norman. "Perceived Risks of Participation in an Epidemiologic Study." *IRB* 15 (No. 1, January/February, 1993): 8-10.

Newell, J. David. "The Case for Deception in Medical Experimentation." *Philosophy in Context* 14 (1984): 51-59.

Novick, Alvin. "At Risk for AIDS: Confidentiality in Research and Surveillance." *IRB* 6 (No. 6, November/December 1984): 10-11.

Novick, Alvin. "Noncompliance in Clinical Trials: I. Subjects." *AIDS and Public Policy Journal* 5 (No. 2, Spring 1990): 94-96.

Passmani, Eugene. "Clinical Trials C Are They Ethical?" *The New England Journal of Medicine* 342 (No. 22, May 30, 1991): 1589-1592.

Poikonen, J.; McCart, G.M.; and Veatch, R.M. "Waivers for Military Use of Investigational Agents." *American Journal of Hospital Pharmacy* 48 (No. 7, July 1991): 1525. Discussion, pp. 1525-9.

Roizen, Ron. "Why I Oppose Drug Company Payment of Physician/Investigators on a Per Patient/Subject Basis." *IRB* 10 (No. 1, January/February 1988): 9-10.

Rosser, Sue V. "Re-Visioning Clinical Research: Gender and the Ethics of Experimental Design." *Hypatia* 4 (No. 2, Summer 1989): 125-139.

Sacks, H.S.; Berrier, J.; Reitman, D.; Ancona-Berk, V.A.; and Chalmers, T.C. "Meta-Analyses of Randomized Controlled Trials." *New England Journal of Medicine* 316 (No. 8, March 18, 1987): 450-455.

Sass, H.M. "Ethical Considerations in Phase I Clinical Trials." *Onkologie* 13 (No. 2, April 1990): 85-88.

Schafer, Arthur. "Commentary: The Randomized Clinical Trial: For Whose Benefit." *IRB* 7 (No. 2, March/April 1985): 4-6.

Schafer, Arthur. "The Ethics of the Randomized Clinical Trials. " *New England Journal of Medicine* 307 (No. 12, September 16, 1982): 719-724.

Schulte, Paul A. "The Epidemiologic Basis for the Notification of Subjects of Cohort Studies." *American Journal of Epidemiology* 121 (No. 3, March 1985): 351-361.

Schuster, Jonathan J. et al. "Ethical Issues in Cooperative Cancer Therapy Trials from a Statistical Viewpoint, I. A General Overview." *American Journal of Pediatric Hematology/Oncology* 7 (No. 1, Spring 1985): 57-63.

Schuster, Jonathan J. et al. "Ethical Issues in Cooperative Cancer Therapy Trials from a Statistical Viewpoint, II. Specific Issues." *American Journal of Pediatric Hematology/Oncology* 7 (No. 1, Spring 1985): 64-70.

Sieber, Joan E. Planning Ethically Responsible Research: A Guide for Students and Internal Review Boards. *Applied Social Research Methods Series*, vol. 31. Newbury Park, CA: Sage Publications, 1992.

Sieber, Joan E., ed. *The Ethics of Social Research: Surveys and Experiments*. New York: Springer-Verlag, 1982.

Sieber, Joan E., ed. *The Ethics of Social Research: Fieldwork, Regulation, and Publication*. New York: Springer-Verlag, 1982.

Soskolne, Colin L. "Scientific and Ethical Conflicts in Cancer Studies Involving Human Subjects." *Women and Health* 11 (No. 3/4, 1986): 197-215.

Spivey, William H. "Informed Consent for Clinical Research in the Emergency Department." *Annals of Emergency Medicine* 18 (No. 7, July 1989): 766-771.

Stanley, Barbara. "An Integration of Ethical and Clinical Considerations in the Use of Placebos." *Psychopharmacology Bulletin* 24 (No. 1, 1988): 18-20.

Stanley, Barbara. "Ethical Considerations in Biological Research on Suicide." In *Psychobiology of Suicidal Behavior*, edited by J. Mann and M. Stanley, pp. 42-46. New York: New York Academy of Sciences, 1986.

Tancredi, Laurence R. ed. *Ethical Issues in Epidemiological Research*. New Brunswick, NJ: Rutgers University Press, 1986.

Thacker, S.B. "Meta-Analysis: A Quantitative Approach to Research Integration." *Journal of the American Medical Association* 259 (No. 11, March 18, 1988): 1685-1689.

U.S. Department of Health and Human Services. Public Health Service. "Privacy Act of 1974: Revision of System of Records." *Federal Register 50* (September 6, 1985): 36491-36494.

U.S. Department of Health and Human Services. Public Health Service. Food and Drug Administration. "Advertising For Study Subjects." *FDA IRB Information Sheets*, February 1989.

U.S. Department of Health and Human Services. Public Health Service. National Institutes of Health. "Policy on Informing Those Tested About HIV Serostatus" [Dear Colleague Letter.] *OPRR Reports*, May 9, 1988.

U.S. Department of Health and Human Services. Public Health Service. National Institutes of Health. "Guidance for Institutional Review Boards for AIDS Studies" [Dear Colleague Letter.] *OPRR Reports*, December 26, 1984.

U.S. Department of Health and Human Services. Public Health Service. National Institutes of Health. *Chemoprevention Clinical Trials: Problems and Solutions*. Bethesda, MD: National Institutes of Health, 1984. NIH Publication No. 85-2715.

U.S. Department of Health and Human Services. Public Health Service. National Institutes of Health. National Cancer Institute. *Investigator's Handbook: A Manual for Participants in Clinical Trials*. Bethesda, MD: National Cancer Institute, 1984.

U.S. Department of Health, Education and Welfare. Food and Drug Administration. *General Considerations for the Clinical Evaluation of Drugs*. Washington, D.C.: U.S. Government Printing Office, 1977. HEW Publication No. (FDA) 77-3040.

U.S. National Research Council. Committee on Models for Biomedical Research. *Models for Biomedical Research: A New Perspective*. Washington, D.C.: National Academy Press, 1985.

VandenBos, Gary R., Guest Editor. "Psychotherapy Research." *American Psychologist* 41 (No. 2, February 1986). The entire volume is devoted to this topic.

Veatch, Robert M. "Drug Research in Humans: The Ethics of Nonrandomized Access." *Clinical Pharmacy* 8 (No. 5, May 1989): 366-370.

Veatch, Robert M. *The Patient as Partner: A Theory of Human-Experimentation Ethics*. Bloomington and Indianapolis, IN: Indiana University Press, 1987. *See* Chapter 13, "Limits on the Right to Privacy: The Ethics of Record Searches and Other Uses of Private Materials."

Veatch, Robert M. "Justice and Research Design: The Case for a Semi-Randomization Clinical Trial." *Clinical Research* 31 (No. 1, February 1983): 12-22.

Veatch, Robert M. "The Patient as Partner: Ethics in Clinical Oncology Research." *The Johns Hopkins Medical Journal* 151 (No. 4, October 1982): 155-161.

Wallace, R. Jay. "Privacy and the Use of Data in Epidemiology." In Ethical Issues in Social Science Research, edited by Tom L. Beauchamp, Ruth R. Faden, R. Jay Wallace, Jr., and LeRoy Walters, pp. 274-291. Baltimore, MD: Johns Hopkins University Press, 1982.

Webb, Eugene J.; Campbell, Donald T.; Schwartz, Richard D.; and Sechrest, Lee. *Unobtrusive Measures: Nonreactive Research in the Social Sciences*. Chicago: Rand McNally, 1966.

Weiss, G.B. "Who Pays for Clinical Research?" *Clinical Research* 27 (1979): 297-299.

World Health Organization, "Potential Use of New Poliomyelitis Vaccines: Memorandum from a WHO Meeting." *Bulletin of the World Health Organization* 68 (No. 5, 1990).

INDEX

C

D

E

I

J

L

M

N

O

P

Q

R

S

T

U

V

W

Y

Z